YOUR MISSING TEETH ARE KILLING YOU!

The Devastating Consequences of Tooth Loss
and the Life-Changing Benefits of Dental Implants

DR. JOSEPH A. GAETA, JR.

ISBN: 978-0-615-60289-9

Public Awareness Publishing
221 Beach Rd PO Box #167
Siesta Key, FL 34242
www.publicawarenesspublishing.com

ACKNOWLEGMENTS

Abundant thanks to my Creator for giving me the inspiration, drive, and passion to make a difference.

To my parents for giving me the upbringing centered on love and service, for helping me come to the realization that we're all in this together, and for always being there with unconditional support in pursuit of my dreams.

To Dr. Carl Misch for the stories he shared of the challenges his grandmother experienced attempting to chew with dentures. And to the Misch International Implant Institute for the guidance, education, and inspiration to relentlessly pursue the science of implant dentistry

This book is also dedicated to all the suffering seniors with dentures who "just get by" while trying to eat. When I started offering public awareness seminars in Florida back in 2001, people would shuffle in with solemn looks, and you could almost "feel" their distress on their faces. After further discovery, it was apparent that many of them were on medication and being treated for numerous diseases: heart, lung, hypertension, etc. Many of them will remain on these medications for the rest of their lives. I came to the realization that I could "fix" their ability to chew with implant dentistry, not like in the medical field where you can't fix the internal organs but only treat symptoms and "manage" their diseases.

I knew that I could help them gain a better quality of life In their twilight years, by securing their dentures with dental implants— so they could smile with confidence and be able to eat foods that they so often turned away because of the inability to chew.

So this book is dedicated to all those suffering denture wearers and people with tooth loss who don't know that there is a better way... They don't have to "just get by" when trying to chew. *Implant dentistry* is the answer.

Extended thanks to those who helped in making this book happen, including:

Lisa M. Rigas, Contributing Editor

Ron White, Graphics Illustrator

CONTENTS

PREFACE

I have been practicing dentistry in southwest Florida for the past twenty-six years. I consider myself blessed to care of seniors, the segment of the population that I consider the salt of the Earth and often the "forgotten segment".

In 1993, I had the good fortune to buy a dental practice from Dr. Harold T. Robbins, a crusty old implant dentist with a dry sense of humor. He was considered a pioneer in implant dentistry. He performed his first dental-implant surgery in 1958, the year I was born!

One morning, Dr. Robbins came to me and said, "Son, if you want to learn implant dentistry and help seniors who can't chew, you better go and get some formal training." He smiled with that familiar, seasoned look and whispered softly under his breath, "Because if you ever go in front of a judge, you can't tell him the old guy with the gray hair taught you how to do implant dentistry!"

This was the beginning of my education and lifelong mission to help suffering denture wearers gain a better quality of life and to chew anything they want with confidence, joy, and a look of total satisfaction. This book is not only for denture wearers but for any person who has experienced tooth loss. It will help you better understand implant dentistry and how you can add *Years to your life and life to your years!*

God Bless, Dr. Gaeta

CHAPTER 1

THE TOOTH-LOSS EPIDEMIC

The world is changing, and people are growing older. In this chapter, I will explain why right now is a crucial moment in dentistry and what it means for your health and happiness.

Americans Are Getting Older

Did you know that in 2010, there were more than forty million people in the United States who were at least sixty-five years old? This number is dramatically higher than just one decade earlier. In the 1960s, less than one-third of the US population was forty-five years old or older, with only 9 percent having reached the age of sixty-five. In 2010, almost 40 percent of the US population was middle-aged or older, and about one person in every eight was at least sixty-five years old.

Americans Are Living Longer

You've heard it on the radio. You've seen it in magazines. The headlines say, "Fifty is the new forty!" This isn't just an exaggeration to sell more magazines. People are actually living longer. What was considered old is now truly middle-aged. This is because the life expectancy of a person born in the 1920s was only fifty-six. But better nutrition and healthcare meant that by the 1980s, life expectancy in the United States was up to the age of seventy. Someone born today is expected to live to be almost eighty.

Older Adults Have Many More Years Ahead of Them

It used to be that a person could only expect to have a few "golden years" after the age of retirement. However, the number of golden years has dramatically increased. Someone who is sixty-five years old can expect to live nineteen more years, and even an eighty-year-old can expect to live nine more years.

The Number of Seniors in the United States Will Continue to Grow

The number of seniors in the United States is going to continue to grow. People are going to continue living longer. Also, the overall population in the United States is expected to increase rapidly. In 2010, there were 40.3 million people in the United States who were sixty-five years old or older. Scientists estimate that by the year 2050, there will be more than eighty-eight million US residents who are sixty-five years old or older. By the time today's children become the adults of tomorrow, the number of seniors will be more than double what it is now.

The Age-Related Tooth-Loss Epidemic

Dental medicine has made tremendous strides. Fluoride added to drinking water and fluoride toothpastes mean that the baby boomer generation will be the first generation in which the majority of the people will maintain their natural teeth over their entire lifetimes. However, oral diseases and dental problems are common among older Americans (age sixty-five years and older) because when they were growing up, community water wasn't fluoridated and there wasn't fluoride toothpaste or mouthwash. Gum disease and cavities are the most frequent causes of tooth loss. Most adults from middle-aged to seniors show signs of gum disease. About one in seven of adults in their late forties and early fifties have severe gum disease.

The seriousness of gum disease increases with age. About one-quarter of seniors aged sixty-five to seventy-four have severe gum disease. Older adults also continue to get cavities on the crowns of their teeth. In addition, they also experience decay on the roots of their teeth as a result of gum recession. Because of this, seniors may get even more new cavities than children do.

Studies have indicated that tooth loss is directly related to age. For adults in their forties and fifties, the number of adults missing all of their natural teeth is only about 5 percent. The number of adults in their sixties and older who are missing all of their natural teeth is 25 percent. Despite progress in dental medicine, one out of twenty middle-aged adults is missing all of his or her natural teeth. And one out of every four seniors is missing all of his or her natural teeth.

How many teeth are lost to this age-related epidemic? A full set of teeth is thirty- two teeth. A 1999 to 2002 survey in the United States found that most adults in their twenties and thirties still had twenty-six or twenty-seven of their teeth. However, the number of teeth rapidly decreases as folks get older. The survey found that adults in their sixties or older had an average of nineteen or twenty natural teeth—twelve to thirteen of their natural teeth were gone!

The first molar is the first permanent teeth we get. Unfortunately, they are also often the first teeth that we lose due to cavities, failed root canals, or tooth fractures. Molars are important teeth for chewing, maintaining the shape of the jaw, and allowing the jaw to close properly during chewing.

CHAPTER 2

THE TRUTH ABOUT DENTURES: DANGERS AND DETRIMENTS

When you re sitting at a table with six other couples, and you go to bite into something, and your dentures slip out, it s rather embarrassing.

Dave

If you currently wear dentures, you can probably identify with Dave's comment. You know firsthand that you can't eat whatever you want while wearing dentures. You've probably had to give up many of your favorite foods. And when you do eat them, you risk pain, embarrassment, or both.

But even if you don't wear dentures, you probably understand that no one really wants to wear them. Dentures are a prosthetic device, like an artificial arm or leg, so obviously they're not preferable to the real thing in almost any circumstance.

Some forty million Americans wear dentures, and most of them will immediately mention discomfort and embarrassment when discussing them.

The truth is that dentures are a detriment to the health of the wearer.

Studies have shown that denture wearers can loose up to 9.8 years off of their life do to the inability to chew their food properly.

Dentures Can Ruin Your Social Life

Dentures have been around since before the days of George Washington's wooden teeth. You would think that with all the advancements modern technology has made over the decades, a comfortable denture would be one of them.

Many seniors who have to wear dentures feel they just have to learn to live with the discomfort, so they just accept that dentures will add aches and pains to the other aches and pains that come with aging. Scientists found that 98 percent of senior patients had sores on their gums from their dentures. Many of them also had something called denture stomatitis, which is an infection in the mouth that is caused by ill- fitting dentures.

Some denture wearers are so embarrassed by their dentures that they refuse to eat in public. They're so uncomfortable eating with their dentures on that they are forced to give up dining with others outside of their homes.

In one study of 873 people forty-five years and older, scientists found that people with full upper dentures were 3.5 times more likely than those who didn't have full dentures to report that they avoided chewing hard things, or that they couldn't eat the foods they liked, or that they avoided eating with others because of chewing problems.

In addition, many denture wearers complain about having trouble speaking. Their words don't come out clearly, the denture gets in the way, and sometimes the dentures slip and move around, which can be embarrassing.

Scientists found that people with full dentures were five times more likely than those who didn't have dentures to report that they avoided laughing and smiling, or they avoided talking, or they had recently felt embarrassed about their mouths.

One of the biggest disadvantages of wearing dentures is the impact on people's social lives. Because of embarrassment or discomfort, dentures are sending normally social, active seniors into isolation. This can lead to depression and other mental health issues that often afflict seniors.

Dangers of Denture Adhesives

Dentures and denture adhesives go together like peanut butter and jelly (something, by the way, you've probably had to give up eating if you actually wear dentures). If you have one, you have the other. Denture wearers have been using the adhesives for years and never thought much about it.

Until now!

Look at this recent report related to the consumer-alert segment the *Today* show aired about the dangers of denture adhesive.

Fixodent, Poligrip, Super Poligrip, and other denture creams have recently been linked to several serious, and **potentially life-threatening**, side effects caused by zinc contained in popular denture creams. Although a small amount of the mineral zinc is necessary for a healthy diet, zinc is toxic when ingested in large amounts and can lead to copper deficiency, which in turn can cause, among other things, peripheral neuropathy. Side effects of a zinc overdose associated with denture cream use may include:

- zinc poisoning (hyperzincemia)
- copper depletion or copper deficiency (hypocupremia)
- neuropathy
- other neurological side effects

In August 2008, a study published in the journal *Neurology* reported on four patients who suffered neuropathy and other neurological denture cream side effects associated with zinc poisoning and copper deficiency. The study, which was conducted by researchers at the University of Texas Southwestern Medical Center in Dallas, noted that while one tube of denture cream should last three to ten weeks, patients in the report were all using at least two tubes of denture cream a week.

It is very distressing that these commonly used creams are potentially life threatening. The last sentence in this article shows just how desperate and frustrated denture wearers can become. The concept of using two whole tubes of adhesive in one week shows the lengths to which a denture wearer will go to force loose dentures to fit firmly and correctly. But in this case, it could be killing them.

Seniors Coming Forward

Across the country, people have been coming forward with stories of becoming weak and even disabled after years of using denture adhesive. They primarily complain of mysterious numbness and weakness in their legs.

Obviously, those claims of weakness and numbness can just be attributed to getting older, as just another one of those inconveniences seniors are forced to endure as the years pile up. But recently, scientists discovered the link between these particular patients' complaints and their dentures. This is a scary revelation.

The Problem with Zinc

As the article indicated, the problem with denture adhesives appears to be the use of the mineral zinc as a bonding agent. To make matters worse, the presence of zinc was never listed on any dental adhesive packaging, at least not at the time.

So what's the problem with zinc? Anyone who's ever taken a vitamin supplement or a high school nutrition class probably knows our bodies need zinc to survive. The problem is that too much zinc definitely falls under the heading "too much of a good thing." In higher doses, zinc can interfere with the absorption of other, equally necessary minerals, such as copper and iron. Without them, our bodies can experience major problems, including numbness and nerve damage.

When Used as Directed

Despite this, the American Dental Association still considers denture adhesives to be safe and has publicly stated that it is not aware of any confirmed cases of adhesives leading to nerve damage. However, seniors (and their attorneys) all over America are saying otherwise.

The denture-adhesive manufacturers maintain that their formulas are safe when used as directed. Those are the key words: "When used as directed."

What exactly does that mean? The instructions included with most tubes of denture adhesive tell users to use just a few small dots of adhesive, strategically placed along the gum line, to keep their dentures securely in place all day long.

You denture wearers out there know that a few dots of adhesive once a day just aren't enough. If you have dentures that don't fit exactly right, or feel less than secure, what else are you going to do? What about denture wearers who, because of discomfort or looseness, take their dentures out and put them back in repeatedly throughout the day? It's a natural impulse to apply more adhesive to keep them in place. After all, you need your dentures to feel secure when you put them back in.

Simply put, many people are probably using more denture adhesive than they are "directed" to. This means that many people are in danger of developing nerve damage.

No Need to Panic   Be Aware

I want to assure you that at this point, there's no need to panic. The problem does not yet appear to be widespread among the entire denture-wearing community. But since the link between denture adhesive and nerve disease was only discovered in 2008, at which time the adhesive manufacturers didn't even list zinc as an ingredient, there may be cases that have not yet been detected.

The denture-adhesive manufacturers are reacting to this problem, including putting disclaimers in their packaging warning against overuse and telling users to talk to their doctors if they are taking zinc supplements. This is all very good advice.

Neurologists now routinely ask many of their patients if they wear, or have worn, dentures. This enables them to immediately address the issue of possible zinc poisoning when they treat them.

Unfortunately, while the progression of symptoms can be stopped when the denture wearer stops using the adhesive, some of the effects, including abnormal limb function, cannot be corrected, even when the mineral imbalance is corrected.

The word to denture wearers, then, is to take action!

Schedule an appointment, get at least two dental implants in the lower jaw, and throw away that potentially toxic denture adhesive once and for all!

Go to **www.secureyourdenturesnow.com** for more information.

Tooth Loss Leads to Bone Loss

If you wear dentures, chances are that when you first got them, they fit pretty well. While they were uncomfortable initially as you got used to them, they probably fit your gums fairly snugly.

However, if you've had those dentures for a while, chances are they don't fit the way they did when they were brand new. There's

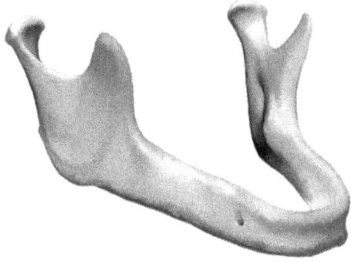

a reason why this happens. It's called bone resorption, which is just a fancy dentist term for bone loss. This is the major danger that comes with tooth loss.

Normally, we think of bone as something that is solid and that doesn't change unless it breaks. In fact, however, our bones are very responsive. Essentially, bones can remodel, depending on the forces that are applied to them. This is why astronauts have to exercise when they are in space. Without the force of gravity, their bones become thinner and weaker. Exercise prevents this.

In order to understand what happens to your bones after you've lost a tooth, you first need to understand how the jawbone works. The upper and lower bones of your jaw actually have two layers: the basal bone and the alveolar bone. The basal bone is the regular part of your skeleton.

But the alveolar bone is specifically formed to hold your teeth. Teeth transmit pressure and tension to the alveolar bone. Chewing stimulates the alveolar bone and is crucial for keeping both the teeth and the underlying bone healthy. When a person loses a tooth, the lack of stimulation to the alveolar bone that had been surrounding the tooth causes the bone to begin shrinking, much like the bones of astronauts shrink if they don't get stimulation from exercisThe shrinking process begins as soon as a tooth is lost or removed. This process has been studied closely, and it is most dramatic during the first year. Immediately after the tooth comes out, a blood clot forms. Two days later, tissue starts to cover the hole. Four days after the tooth was lost, the body starts to break down the ridge in the bone where the tooth used to be. By about a month later, that place in the jaw is only about two-thirds as tall as it had been when there was a tooth.

To better understand this concept and see a free video of this serious consequence of tooth loss, please visit

www.yourmissingteetharekillingyou.com.

Progression of Bone Full Dentition

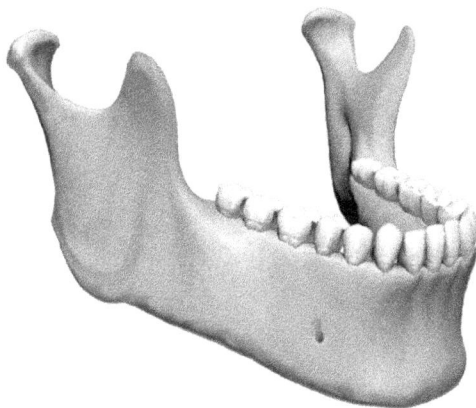

Tooth
Loss

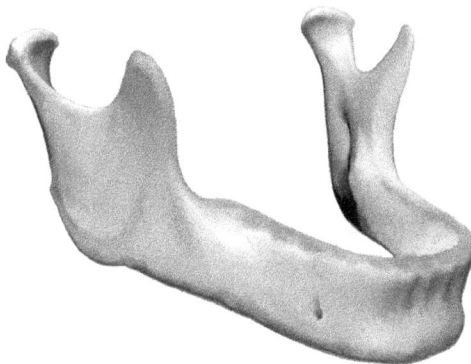

Tooth and
Bone Loss

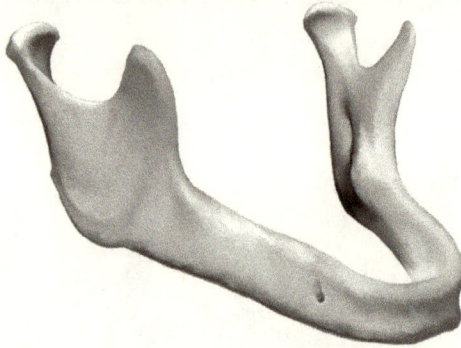

More Bone Loss

It's not just the bone that's affected—it's the gum tissue, too. As the bones in a person's jaw lose width and height, the attached gum tissue gradually becomes thinner. Therefore, a person may have sore spots and feel more discomfort under his or her dentures. If a person has lost many teeth, his or her tongue often enlarges to fill the now-empty space. At the same time, people start using their tongues to keep their dentures from moving. The tongue may take a more active role in the chewing process, and this leads to the dentures feeling less stable.

As long as there are teeth missing, the shrinkage of the jawbone is a lifelong, irreversible problem. You will continue to loose bone for the rest of your life unless you STOP THE BONELOSS WITH DENTAL IMPLANTS!!

After about three months, almost a quarter of the bone is gone. One-third of the bone is gone by six months. In that first year after the loss of a tooth, the loss of bone is approximately ten times more than it is in the following years.

Tooth Loss, Bone Loss, and Premature Aging

Your teeth support the lower third of your face. Losing teeth can have a dramatic impact on your appearance. Without a tooth taking up the space next to them, any teeth that regularly come in contact with that tooth start to shift into the empty space. Even the overall height of your face can shrink as your jawbones collapse.

This explains why, if you've been wearing dentures for a while, they probably don't fit like they used to. For one thing, the lower jaw begins losing bone at a faster rate than the upper jaw. This leads to the appearance of a shrinking jawline. The lower jaw also begins to protrude out farther than the upper jaw. Your dentures no longer fit because your jaw isn't the same shape it was back when you were fitted for them in the first place.

The Wicked Witch

Sometimes a cartoon can highlight something that happens in real life. For example, the cartoon version of a wicked witch highlights what actually does happen with tooth loss and bone loss. The loss of bone in the upper jaw means that the upper lip seems to disappear. The lack of upper lip makes the nose seem more prominent. The lack of teeth and bone on the lower part of the jaw makes the chin rotate forward and stick out.

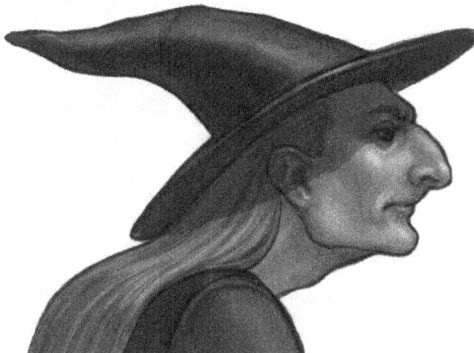

The lips—especially the upper lip—are thin. There is a deepening of the vertical wrinkles around the mouth, and the person seems to frown when her mouth is closed. The muscles around the lips either contract or they collapse, leading to deeper wrinkles in the mouth area. And while some wrinkles are a normal part of aging, the loss of tooth and bone makes the wrinkles deeper. Weak, sagging muscles in the lower part of your face contribute to jowls and what's known as a "witch's chin."

Progression of the Premature Aging Effects of Bone Loss as a Consequence of Tooth Loss

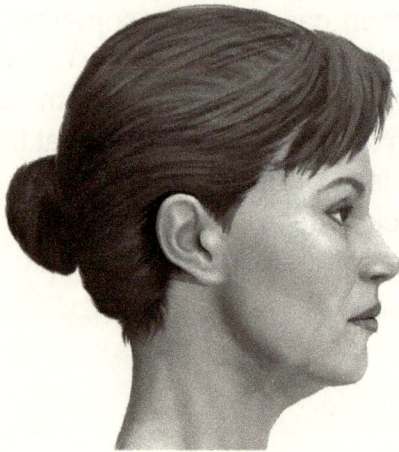

Tooth Loss

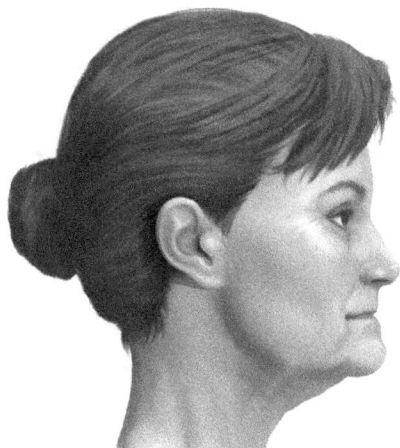

Tooth Loss with Bone Loss

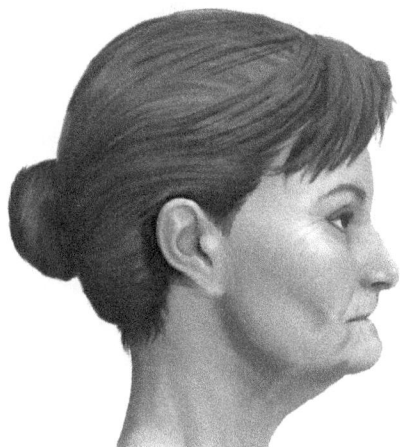

Tooth Loss with Additional Bone Loss

YOUR MISSING TEETH ARE KILLING YOU!

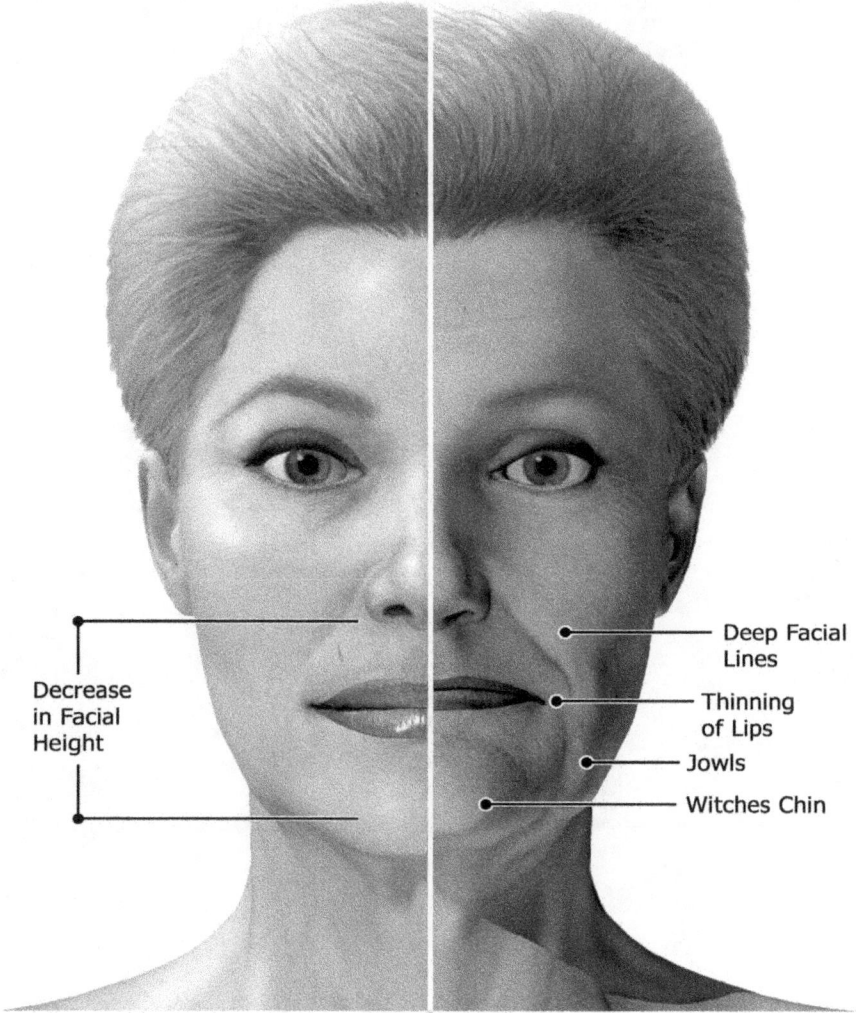

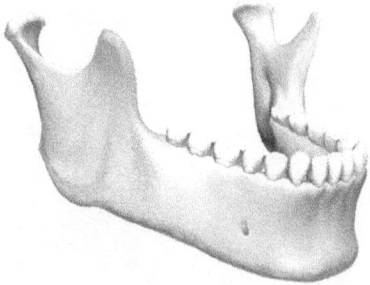

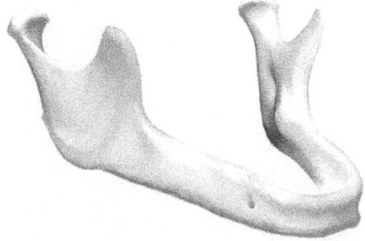

Decrease in Facial Height

Deep Facial Lines

Thinning of Lips

Jowls

Witches Chin

The image of a wicked witch is not far from the truth of what actually happens when teeth and bone are lost. You may have begun noticing changes that make it seem like your face is aging much faster than the rest of your body—and certainly aging much faster than you feel.

Even if you wear dentures, there is nothing you can do to stop the bone-loss process. The dentures sitting on top of your gums can maintain some of your facial form. But your jawbone needs stimulation to maintain its shape, density, and strength. Full dentures, partial dentures, and the false tooth or teeth in the center of a bridge do not attach directly to your bone. Therefore, they can't stimulate your jawbone to stop it from shrinking.

Dentistry for seniors used to focus on straightforward treatments like dentures because seniors weren't expected to live the long, vital lives that they do now. However, now that life expectancies are longer, dental treatments that will last longer are needed, too.

To better understand the physical effects of tooth loss, please visit **www.yourmissingteetharekillingyou.com** for a free video, which details this serious consequence of tooth loss.

Dentures Don t Help Because They Restrict Your Diet
The Role of Bite Force

The problem is bite force. When you had your natural teeth, the force of your bite was an average—at your molars, where you do most of your chewing, bite force is 150 to 250 psi. But the maximum bite force of the average denture wearer is less than 50 psi—and after wearing dentures for over fifteen years their bite force can be reduced to only 5.6 psi! Meaning at the best, it's 60 percent lower than it used to be. You can understand why eating with dentures is so difficult. You just don't have the power.

When you can't chew very well, a few things happen. You eat fewer fruits and vegetables because they require chewing. You experience gastrointestinal disorders from food that isn't broken up properly. It can even be hard to swallow.

> To better understand the effects of tooth loss on bite force, please visit **www.yourmissingteetharekillingyou.com** for a free video, which details this serious consequence.

Lack of Proper Nutrition

It stands to reason that when people aren't eating the nutritious foods that they once loved, their nutrient intake will suffer. This is due to discomfort and pain and also to the inability to chew correctly. The very foods that the body needs for proper nutrition are the very foods that are now impossible for denture wearers to eat. This could include lean meats, whole grains, fruits, and vegetables. The problem is that an ideal diet is made up of a lot of foods that require chewing. And the very act of chewing has now become marginalized due to the loss of bite force.

We all know what kind of diet we're supposed to be eating to be at our best—a diet made up of lean meats, whole grains, fruits, and vegetables. The problem is that an ideal diet is made up of a lot of foods that require chewing.

Body Weight and Mortality

Many people who wear dentures end up losing too much weight. Some people end up gaining weight because they're unable to eat fruits and vegetables. A study of 629 seniors in Britain illustrated this phenomenon. Scientists found that people with fewer than ten teeth were four times as likely to be underweight than those who had eleven or more teeth. Meanwhile, people with fewer than twenty-one natural teeth were more than three times as likely to be obese than seniors who still had twenty-one natural teeth or more.

Doctors conducted a study of 322 veterans who had health problems. These veterans had just been discharged from the hospital, and the average veteran was seventy-six years old. Before patients left the hospital, doctors checked their nutritional status, particularly as it related to protein.

Over the next six years, the doctors found that nutrition mattered more for longevity than whether a person had had heart failure, more than whether the person was living on his or her own or in a nursing home, and even more than age.

Specifically, doctors checked who had low protein levels and who was underweight to figure out the level of nutrition risk. They used the body mass index to decide if a person was underweight. The idea is that once a person leaves the hospital, whatever health condition brought them to the hospital is more or less resolved. However, having poor nutrition levels meant having a higher risk of health problems. It's important to remember that these patients were considered the "frail elderly."

If a patient had a basically normal protein level and a normal body mass index, then he was considered to be low risk. On average, this type of person survived for almost four and a half years after leaving the hospital. On the other hand, if a person had low protein levels and was underweight, then he was considered to be high risk. This type of veteran survived for only about one year after leaving the VA hospital.

It's so sad. For seniors who don't get enough nutrition when they need it most, their lives may be tragically cut short.

Teeth and Life Span

In 1984, four dental scientists in Denmark set out to identify the early signs of accelerated aging. Their thinking was that by determining the early signs and addressing them, they could prevent some disability. They looked closely at tooth loss. They studied the health of 573 people who were in their seventies and kept track of them up to 2006. These scientists even took into account different factors like income, health conditions like high blood pressure, and how tired or physically active each person was.

They found that by the age of seventy-five, a person who had lost all of his or her teeth was almost three times more likely to be physically disabled than a person with twenty or more teeth. Even more startling that was that someone with no teeth had a 265 percent higher risk of dying sooner than a person who still had teeth.

 The study showed that the average person who had no natural teeth lived for about 11.5 more years after the study began. Meanwhile, the average person who had twenty or more teeth lived for about 17.5 more years.

In other words, teeth can add about six years to your life!

Making It from Age Seventy to Age Eighty in Italy

Researchers from Italy did a study of 1,124 people in their early seventies who were all city dwellers and healthy enough to live at home. These researchers wanted to see if there were differences among three groups: those who had enough natural teeth (at least sixteen of them), those who didn't have enough natural teeth (fewer than sixteen), and those who wore some kind of dentures (whether removable or fixed, partial or complete).

The results were rather interesting. First, both the seniors with an adequate number of natural teeth and the seniors who wore dentures were able to complete their day-to-day activities.

But people with enough natural teeth were more likely to say that they had satisfying social relationships than either people with dentures or the people who had few teeth. Also, people with enough teeth were less likely to need health services than either the people who wore dentures or the people who didn't have enough teeth.

Ten years after the first study, the researchers checked government records to see what had happened to the people they had studied. They found out that over half of the people who had participated in the study were still alive.

However, there were differences in the numbers of people who had survived in each group. Of seniors who had enough natural teeth, 67 percent were still alive. Of the seniors who had dentures, 55 percent were still alive. For the people who did not have enough teeth and were not using any type of dentures, 52 percent were still alive. In other words, for every one hundred people with natural teeth who survived the ten years, only seventy-four people with dentures also survived, and only sixty-seven people who had neither dentures nor enough teeth survived.

Making It from Age 81 to Age 108 in California

At Leisure World retirement community in California, 5,611 older adults were studied for an average of nine years. These were well-educated, upper-middle-class people with an average age of 81. This study started in 1992, and the researchers took into account all the things you might think would affect longevity, including activity level, whether the seniors had other ailments, and whether they smoked or drank. Some of the seniors were very healthy—one person even lived to be 108!

This study showed that teeth matter a lot for longevity. In this study, the researchers looked specifically at a person's risk of dying. Unfortunately, individuals with no teeth (even those who wore dentures) had a 30 percent higher risk of death compared with the seniors who had twenty or more natural teeth. In most all (90 percent) of the seniors who had fewer than sixteen teeth had dentures that they could wear. Whether they live in Italy or in the United States, seniors with teeth tend to live longer.

> To better understand the effects of tooth loss on bite force, please visit **www.yourmissingteetharekillingyou.com** for a free video, which details this serious consequence.

Can Your Dentures Actually Kill You?

Yes, I admit, it sounds dramatic. Unfortunately, it's also true—at least if you believe the National Institute of Health. After a long-term study, they concluded that patients who maintain most or all of their natural teeth, have missing teeth replaced by fixed bridgework, or have teeth supported by dental implants live longer than patients who wear removable dentures or partials.

How much longer? How about 9.8 years longer? In other words, wearing dentures can actually take about 10 years off your life!

How can this happen? How can a simple appliance that's been around forever and is supposed to help you put you in danger?

The answer is simple. And it's all about eating. Seniors, who need good nutrition to remain strong and healthy, don't get the calories or the nutrients they need when they wear dentures. This goes on to the point where they are being robbed of almost ten years of their lives.

Luckily, there is something you can do to get those years back. You can replace your dentures with dental implants.

Not All Bad News

In this chapter I have presented some of the dangers and detriments that denture wearers face. You may have considered some of these factors, but perhaps you haven't heard of some of them. Chances are you did not know that dentures are one of the leading contributors to premature aging.

I believe that dentures lead to a worse quality of life—and that's something that people don't have to endure.

In the following chapters, I will offer a detailed look at dental implants so that you will better understand why they offer a safe and satisfying alternative to dentures!

First, though, take a look at these two stories from patients of mine. One story is from my own mother, Josephine Gaeta. Yes, my mother is my patient, as was my father, Joseph, Sr., until his recent passing.

And then we have Loretta's exciting story! Loretta's dentures were literally making her sick. But there's a happy ending.

Josephine's Story

"I have had a full set of dentures for many years. They were never comfortable, especially the bottom set. They moved around and bothered me a lot. I always had to take them out and clean them every time I ate. That was such a bother.

"So, about fifteen years ago, I had four implants in my bottom jaw. These are used to firm up the dentures. It helps them stay in place. It made such a difference.

"Now they stay in place. They don't move around, and I don't have to take them out as often. That makes such a difference for me.

"My husband passed away about a year ago. We'd been married fifty-eight years!

"I'm thankful I had the implants done, and my future goal is to eventually get rid of the upper denture and have all implants put in. I'd like to know what it's like to have the roof of my mouth back again!"

* * *

Loretta's Story

"I had several teeth missing and had a horrible partial bridge. My gums were in extremely poor condition, with many bad pockets. Because of the dentures, I could not chew or swallow my food properly; sometimes my food was half chewed when I swallowed. This led to poor eating habits so bad I was on stomach medications for years.

"I was extremely self-conscious when eating out. I avoided talking at restaurants and was always afraid that food particles were hooked to my partial. So I was always going to the restroom to clean and check my teeth. This was very embarrassing and made me feel self-conscious.

"A friend of mine had started with implants, and I went with him to drive him home. My friend kept after me to get implants because he knew from his own experience how uncomfortable I was with my dental plates. But I hate going to the dentist due to very bad past experiences, both as a child and as an adult. So I was a nervous wreck about it. But the process went smoothly, and trust me — as a former coward — I felt nothing! I was overwhelmed the first time I saw my new smile. No more hooks connected to my teeth! It was wonderful and exciting. My recovery took about one and a half days. I had some bruising, which I was informed would be normal, and took Ibuprofen for the discomfort while using an ice pack to keep any swelling down.

"I even loved my temporary teeth. They threw my old metal palate-partial denture away! I was able to eat for the first time in years with nothing covering my palate and was able to chew and swallow all foods without embarrassment, with no more food sticking to my bridgework.

"My life today is great. I smile a lot more, I feel more confident, and I eat and chew all foods, a whole lot! I would tell anyone who is considering dental implant surgery, don't waste anymore time thinking about it. If you want to feel and look better and want to eat all foods, do it."

* * *

CHAPTER 3

DENTISTS AND THEIR PATIENTS

What I really liked about this whole experience was that the surgical phase and the restorative phase were approached together, so the implant and the restorative dentistry were done at one place.

Jem

Have you ever met anyone who just loved to go to the dentist? Does anyone get pleasure from having a cavity filled or getting a root canal? I doubt it.

As a child, I was petrified to go to the dentist. I was a chubby, little Italian kid who loved to eat. (All Italians love to eat.) For that reason I had a whole slew of cavities, and I frequently went to the dentist, where I always had to have something done.

Obviously, the lack of sophisticated technology contributed to the unpleasant experience of going to the dentist. I was terrified, and I could always feel the drill.

I'll never forget one day I had to go to the dentist to have an abscess taken care of, and I was so frightened that I hid under the dentist's desk. Funny, though, that I always knew that I wanted to be a dentist.

My First Mentor

I graduated from Creighton University Dental School in 1986, and I worked in a clinic in Omaha, Nebraska, for a couple of years. I was fortunate to work with a wonderful mentor whose name was Jim Demman.

This wonderful man taught me the three reasons why people are reluctant to go to the dentist. I've never forgotten them:

1. Fear
2. Money
3. Low dental IQ. (In other words, most people are generally ignorant of many of the aspects of dentistry. Dr. Demman was also a big proponent of patient education.)

Conscious Sedation

I still use many of Dr. Demman's strategies in my practice today. I use what is called conscious sedation. With conscious sedation, a couple of drugs are administered with an IV, after which the patient responds to verbal stimulation but feels and remembers nothing! The drugs make you amnesic. It's a wonderful drug, and it's very very safe (it's the same type of medication that is administered during a colonocoscopy procedure). The morbidity rate (death rate) is one in 858,000.

Over the course of my career, I have witnessed conscious sedation absolutely and completely alter the way my patients feel about visiting the dentist. Once you address their fear, gain their trust, and perform a procedure with sedation, it changes their entire perspective on how comforting and enjoyable a dental procedure can actually be.

Fear with Good Reason

Occasionally, patients come to me who have every reason to be reluctant about going to a dentist. Wayne T., age fifty, suffers from cerebral palsy and must use a wheelchair. Living in a colder climate is extremely difficult for someone like Wayne, so he decided to move from his home in Rock Island, Illinois, to Florida. He said he was tired of getting cabin fever every winter. His mother and stepfather, Rosemary and Patrick Hardy, helped him make the move.

Once they arrived in Florida, they ate out in a restaurant. While eating, Wayne had a tooth fall out. As Rosemary says, "This wasn't the first time he'd had a tooth fall out, so we knew it was time. We had to do something. It was time to go to the dentist."

Wayne protested. Just like most folks, he dreaded the thought of going to the dentist, but for someone in a wheelchair, that fear is greatly intensified. After asking around, someone recommended that they consult with me.

Because of our use of conscious sedation, Wayne had absolutely no stress. Everything was taken care of in one visit, including taking out the top teeth and even performing some surgical processes on the bottom teeth. All told, it took about four hours, during which Wayne was perfectly comfortable, calm, and rested.

Because of the limited range of motion in Wayne's hands and arms, having a set of dentures would be out of the question. He would never be able to take them in and out on a daily basis.

Patrick, a denture wearer himself and familiar with the challenges they can bring, was in total agreement. Implants then became the most feasible answer.

Diane's Story

"I'm an author. I'm in the middle of completing the third book in my mystery series about Sir Arthur Conan Doyle. So I spend some time in front of the public at book signings and events.

"My problem was that I had a great fear of dentists. Believe it or not, years ago in Chicago, I had Kim N.'s dentist, and I didn't like him. He never gave me any Novocain or anything. One time when he was doing a filling, I nearly jumped out of a chair, and he said, "Oh, that's your nerve!"

"That is probably the basis for my fears.

"And I have a sensitive mouth on top of all that. I think most people who have sensitive mouths really dislike dental work.

"I never had braces or anything, so I had irregular teeth and an irregular bite. Beyond that, people couldn't tell there was anything wrong with me. But for me it was a health problem. When my husband and I moved to Florida, I could not find a dentist. I tried two dentists and didn't like either of them, so I had a period of not getting good dental care. I was afraid that my gums were deteriorating and that I would be losing a lot of teeth. I wanted to get that taken care of, and I didn't want dentures.

"My dentist discussed implants with me. He kept his promise that he was very conscious of people who had dental fears, and his staff was also conscious of that. They treated me very well. No other dentist who I'd been to considered the entire dental overview of my mouth and what I was going to be needing and wanting in the future. When he saw what my problems were, he came up with a creative solution that I really liked.

"He worked very hard to save whatever teeth he could save. He had to be extremely clever with what he did. There was one tooth that he did an implant for that he had to kind of rotate just right to make sure that my bite was right.

"I have implants on both the top and the bottom. They tell you exactly what is going to be happening when, and in the meantime, when you don't have some of your implants yet, they give you temporary teeth so you're able to function completely normally.

"I didn't have all of my implants in, but I went on a book-signing tour with my temporary teeth, and everything was fine. They're very normal, very natural looking. My new smile is better than my old smile. It's so much better. I have the kind of smile I would have had if I had braces.

"Today I feel better, and I think I look better. It is a process. It isn't like going in and getting the dentures in just one day, but it is definitely worth it. They feel like your regular teeth. Implant dentistry, if done properly, is a miracle."

* * *

Jems's Story

"After a baseball accident when I was eighteen years old, I was told I needed two root canals and then crowns to fix the damage. At the time, the choice was to lose my front teeth or have them fixed. It was a no-brainer. I had them fixed!

"Over the years, these two teeth gave me so many problems that I often wished that I had had them removed and had dealt with a bridge. I had the root canals and the crowns redone. Then the apex of the tooth was removed due to infection and had to be filled from the root tip. This was a surgical procedure, and I can honestly say that it was not a fun day!

"Remember, it was not just one tooth I was dealing with, but two. It was the one in the front and one on the side. So usually, my mouth was sore, and every problem was multiplied by two. Through the years, it was an ongoing struggle to keep it pain-free and to maintain my smile.

"Then one day I bit into a burger, and the front tooth just snapped off. The bad news was that everything was lost, and it could not be restored. The good news was that by cleaning everything out, it was ideal for a dental implant. I made that decision, and it turned out to be the right one. For the first time in years, this area was pain-free. Everything looked and felt great!

"Now my only concern was the tooth on the side since it was still problematic! Then one day the tooth flared up. I was in some serious pain! I went to my local dentist, who took a digital x-ray and detected a root fracture. In addition, he informed me that there was a low-grade infection that ate away most of the bone. Attached to the root tip were a granulation tissue and a cystic sac that needed to be removed immediately. This was all bad news!

"Then he told me that he wanted me to see an implant dentist. He told me that any dental work of this nature was referred over to him, and he reassured me that he was an expert in this area of dentistry, and if anyone could fix this problem with a lasting result, he would be the one.

"He informed me that the fractured tooth would have to be removed. All the infection, scar tissue, and the cyst would have to be removed, after which he would graft bone into the area. Once the bone graft took and everything was healthy again (which would be four to five months), he would place an implant.

"He explained that the implant would need four months to take hold and become stable; then he would put a crown in place. The dentist said that while he couldn't give a 100 percent guarantee that everything would work according to this plan, he felt that given my situation and my health, he was 99 percent sure it would be successful.

"At this point, my only fear was that I would have to go around with a gap in my smile or wear some removable device that would be embarrassing. He told me not to worry about that, because he guaranteed that I would never have to go without a tooth in that area. He said that I would have a great-looking tooth that was going to be temporarily placed while healing took place. This was definitely good enough for me! I went for it.

"Everything went according to plan, and today I am pain-free, and I can eat anything I want. Everything looks great and feels great. What I really liked about this whole experience was that the dentist resolved the surgical phase in a way that set up the restorative phase, because he is trained to do all aspects of implant and restorative dentistry."

* * *

CHAPTER 4

THE HISTORY OF DENTAL IMPLANTS

Getting implants was marvelous   just the best decision I ever made. I was excited the day I could eat pizza again   and all my other dreamy foods!

Walter

Although you may think of dental implants as a modern invention, in fact they have been around for centuries!

Mayans Had the Right Idea

I'm almost positive that no one would associate dental implants with 600 AD. In fact, they might go back even further. However, 600 AD is the earliest physical evidence we have of the existence of dental implants.

This groundbreaking discovery came in 1931, when a team of archeologists were on a dig in Honduras at an ancient Mayan burial site. The team unearthed what appeared to be a large section of the mandible, or lower jaw, of a woman in her twenties. This alone was a pretty amazing find.

But even more amazing was that in her lower jaw, in the spots where three teeth were missing, three tooth-shaped pieces of shell had been inserted. And some nineteen hundred years later, they were still there!

The scientists who investigated the find originally assumed that the shells were just placed there as decoration when the woman was buried, perhaps to make her "whole" again in the afterlife. After all, the ancient Egyptians did the same thing with their dead.

Scientific Breakthrough

The scientific community continued to believe that this Mayan jaw was just another jaw—albeit a well-decorated one—for four more decades. They had no idea that what they had found was actually the earliest evidence of a genuine scientific breakthrough.

But in Brazil in 1970, a dental professor named Amadeo Bobbio had other ideas about the mysterious mandible. He wondered if perhaps there was another reason that the shell "teeth" had survived along with the jaw.

He examined the mandible more closely, looking inside the fossil with a series of radiographs, which are basically a kind of x-ray. What he found was truly remarkable.

New bone had formed around the three pieces of shell, locking them in place, much like natural teeth. This means that they were placed in the woman's jaw when she was still alive, and her body accepted them; at least the bone aspect of her body did. In other words, Bobbio had discovered the first known evidence of dental implants.

So even back in 600 AD, people understood the value of their teeth and the need to preserve them. They knew that the best replacement for a lost tooth was another tooth anchored in the jaw.

The Search for a Viable Tooth Replacement

And the ancient Mayans weren't alone. The search for a viable replacement for lost teeth was going on in other places around the world during ancient times. Ancient dentists tried using materials ranging from gold to silver to carbon fiber to fill in for teeth that were lost.

They even tried using teeth extracted from other people's mouths, which led to some pretty nasty consequences. There were no antirejection drugs in those days, so teeth from other people's mouths were treated as invading organisms by their new bodies and rejected. Serious infections were also known to occur.

Finding a dental implant that was both safe and effective just wasn't possible, given the level of technology at the time. This is probably why the idea of dentures—which basically amounts to sticking the replacement teeth on top of the gums rather than trying to make them part of the jaw like natural teeth—grew in popularity. They were the simplest and most basic solution to the problem of tooth loss. But they were also, by no means, the best one.

The search for an alternative continued.

Titanium Enters the Picture

The breakthrough began in the late 1950s at England's Cambridge University. A team was researching the flow of blood in vivo, which to everyone outside the scientific community simply means within a living organism. Somehow, this led to this particular team using the metal titanium to construct a small chamber that was then embedded into the ears of rabbits.

A Swedish orthopedic surgeon named P-I Brånemark discovered the link. In 1952, while the Cambridge team was still studying blood flow, he was conducting his own study of how bones heal and regenerate. And for some reason, he also opted to test his theories on rabbits.

Brånemark adapted the titanium "rabbit ear chamber" from the Cambridge team to use in rabbit legs, to help heal injured bones.

But when he tried to get those titanium chambers out of the rabbit legs to study what had happened to them, he found that they were stuck.

Brånemark discovered that the bone had grown so close to the titanium tubes that it had basically stuck to the metal and actually integrated it into the rabbits' legs. Further study, on both people and animals, proved Brånemark's theory that titanium was a unique and very viable substitute for bone.

He called his discovery of bone's nearly seamless interaction and acceptance of titanium "osseointegration"—because "osseo" means "bone," and we all know what "integration" means. The titanium had integrated into the bone.

Tooth Loss the Best Test

As an orthopedist, Brånemark's original intention for his discovery was to find ways to use titanium in knee and hip surgery, something that is commonly done today. But he needed subjects to test his theory on, and hip and knee surgery could be, at the time, a very invasive process with a long healing time.

He found a better pool of test subjects in people who had suffered tooth loss. The procedure to test titanium in the jawbone was far less invasive.

So in 1965, Brånemark, now a professor of anatomy at Gothenburg University in Sweden, placed the very first titanium dental implant into his very first human volunteer, a Swedish man named Gösta Larsson (who, incidentally, lived forty more years, until 2005).

At the same time, US scientists were conducting their own research and filed for a US patent for titanium dental implants in 1969. Meanwhile, Brånemark continued to publish studies on his discovery and ultimately went into a commercial partnership with a Swedish company, now called Nobel Industries, to continue to develop state-of-the-art implants.

Millions of Implants Later

Since the 1960s, the majority of all dental implants have been made of titanium. More than seven million of Brånemark's implants have been placed, with hundreds of other companies worldwide also manufacturing dental implants. For over forty years, they have reigned as one of the most successful technological advances ever in the field of dentistry.

Of course, scientists are always on the lookout for something newer, better, easier, and/or cheaper. While titanium implants have been and still are stunningly successful, researchers are still working to develop the next big thing in implant technology.

Currently, some of the most promising research in the field of dental implantology is focusing on a ceramic-type material called zirconia, which comes from the metal zirconium. Since zirconium is close to titanium, the hope is that it will behave in much the same way as titanium implants. And since zirconia is a ceramic, it will create one-piece implants that simulate natural teeth all the way down to the roots.

Studies are still being done as to the long-term viability of implants made of zirconia, so for now, titanium is still widely used.

Choosing implants was definitely the way to go for both Walter and Steve. Here are their stories:

Walter's Story

"I started about ten years ago, and I got implants over about a year and a half. I am now sixty-seven, so it would be safe to say I was fifty-eight. I was missing one or two teeth, had been missing them for years. My teeth weren't unhealthy, but they just looked like crap. I had been missing one or two teeth for years, and the ones left were crooked and full of fillings and things like that.

"I grew up healthy but poor. Back then, teeth weren't a priority like they are today. We were lucky if we got to see a dentist once a year.

"I was in sales, my mouth was always in front of a potential customer, and I didn't have a great smile. I was self-conscious, and I wasn't happy with the way I looked. I was not afraid to smile, but I wasn't real comfortable. I would catch myself putting my hand over my mouth. Not that my teeth were nasty and green. I always had good hygiene, but just poor teeth.

"Getting implants was marvelous—just the best decision I ever made. What a difference. After the implants, I just felt more secure—self-esteem, I guess.

"I actually don't know how many of my teeth were replaced with implants, probably five or six, but I just don't know. When I first had them done I would get compliments from strangers and people I knew, and I still get compliments ten years later.

"The dentist worked with me to make it affordable. When I could afford to lay out x number of dollars, I would have one done or two done.

"The one day I remember the most clearly was after I finished up, I walked into a Home Depot on a Sunday morning, dressed in grubbies and covered with sawdust. And they have a greeter at the front door, and she said, 'Wow you have a beautiful smile, and look at those teeth!'

"I don't know, maybe she was flirting, but I felt very comfortable. I made sure I was smiling to make sure she could see my teeth. And she kept going, 'I can't get over it. At your age your teeth look beautiful.'

"I still work part-time. I sell wine for a living, and when you sell wine you spend a lot of time with a customer. You spend a lot of time to close a sale, sometimes two or three meetings, and two and three hours long; your mouth is in front of everybody constantly. You're also tasting wine with people. Wine is very staining, and the implants are not affected as much as regular teeth.

"If you're thinking of getting implants, my advice is to do research. Go to the Internet. There are some good blogs. I don't recall reading anything negative. And number two, move forward; don't put it off. There's no reason to put it off, except maybe financial. But even then, you need to ask yourself, if an implant is a thousand dollars, what is that worth? Is it worth a sale? Honestly, I wish I had it done twenty years earlier. Maybe I didn't need it then, but it gave me the kind of smile I never had when I was younger."

* * *

Steve's Story

"Growing up I had a number of bad experiences with dentists. By the time I was in my twenties and experienced a good dentist, I was surprised that they actually used Novocain to deaden the area being worked on.

"For the most part, dentists just kept filling and filling, until one dentist looked at one of my teeth and remarked, 'That isn't even a tooth anymore.' When I looked in the mirror, it looked more like a skull, because of so much work that had been done. It was also painful to chew, and any cold liquids caused excruciating pain.

"I moved to Florida from New England. I'm fifty-eight now, and I had the work done in 2008. I appreciated the fact that I didn't have to keep going to another specialist to get part of the work done. Everything took place in one office, and a great deal of the work was done in one sitting. Because I had such a fear from all my childhood experiences, it's wonderful now to go to the dentist and not be afraid.

"I admit that I heal rather slowly. I'm a smoker and a coffee drinker, and I'm sure that has something to do with it. All told, the entire process took about nine months. I was excited the day I could eat pizza again—and all my other dreamy foods!

"Now that my teeth are fixed and the implants in place, I feel better overall. It's like I have a new sense of well-being. I am convinced that dental health affects all the other parts of our bodies, and it's a shame that it does not receive the attention it deserves. I call dental health the 'gateway to the body.' Now I have no pain chewing. I look better and feel better. My confidence is restored.

"I definitely would recommend getting implants and am so thankful I took that step. While it may be rather expensive, I take into consideration that these new teeth are going to last me an entire lifetime."

* * *

CHAPTER 5

UNDERSTANDING DENTAL IMPLANTS

Today, I m eating better and living better and am more self-confident. I'm friendlier, and being friendlier, you accumulate more friends   Don t hesitate, just have it done. You ll never, never be sorry.

Herman

In this chapter, I will show you how dental implants work and how they can help you restore your smile and your self-confidence.

Dental implants are a viable, safe, and effective alternative to dentures that will dramatically improve your quality of life, from the way you look to the way you feel.

Just Like Natural Teeth

Created from medical-grade titanium (no different from a hip or a knee implant—in fact it's the same type of titanium!), stronger than natural teeth, a dental implant is a replacement for a natural tooth that is actually anchored into your jaw just like your real teeth are. Dental implants behave just like natural teeth. They stay in your mouth permanently, not in a glass next to the bathroom sink like Grandpa's dentures. They give you the same strong bite you had when you had your natural teeth, which means you can eat crunchy apples, corn on the cob, steaks, sandwiches, *anything your heart desires!*

Even better, you'll be able to show the world a big, beautiful smile, no matter what your age. You'll enjoy the freedom of never worrying about your teeth—beyond basic oral hygiene, of course—ever again. And you'll enjoy the renewed confidence that only a great smile can provide.

The bottom line is that dental implants offer seniors an improved quality of life that has to be experienced to be believed. Having implants can be life changing.

It s Really No Mystery

You may be wondering why more people aren't getting implants if they are so good. For many people, implants are still a big mystery. Some people think they're complicated or expensive.

The Just Getting By Syndrome

For many seniors, not knowing is an excuse to keep not doing anything. It's an excuse to keep things the way they are. If Grandpa lived with dentures, why shouldn't they? This is what I call the "Just Getting By" Syndrome.

And that's what I am here to change. People don't have to suffer the "Just Getting By" Syndrome.

The Part You Can t See

A dental implant only stands in for the part of the tooth you don't see, the artificial tooth root. A titanium screw anchors a tooth to your jawbone. It's really nothing more than a titanium screw that is surgically implanted into the jawbone.

Obviously, having a mouth full of titanium screws is not what you think of when you imagine a "just like new" replacement for your natural teeth. But that titanium screw is only the beginning. It's the foundation for rebuilding your big, beautiful smile.

This is because the metal used to make dental implants is titanium—a substance that reacts very favorably to your natural bone. Once the implant is placed in your jawbone, that jawbone, which is alive, accepts the titanium as a natural part of the body. A process called osseointegration takes place, during which the natural bone around the implant grows around the titanium screw, locking it into place, making the implant an actual part of your jaw, just like a natural tooth root. Structurally and functionally, your implants are connected to your body, and they work just like a part of your body. They also help to maintain the natural shape of your jaw by stopping bone loss and even stimulating new bone growth.

The Part You Can See

As I mentioned before, implants are only half of the story.

The other half is what goes on top of them: beautiful, glorious, and functional teeth.

Okay, they're not real teeth. But it's nearly impossible to tell the difference.

One of the best things about dental implants is that they are made in a variety of sizes and types, to accommodate just about any tooth-replacement situation. They can be configured to support all kinds of replacement teeth, from a single missing tooth to an entire mouthful.

Single Missing Tooth

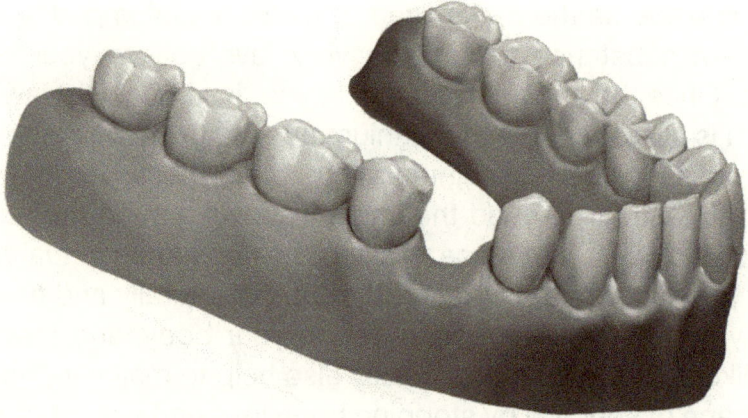

Single Tooth Dental Implant

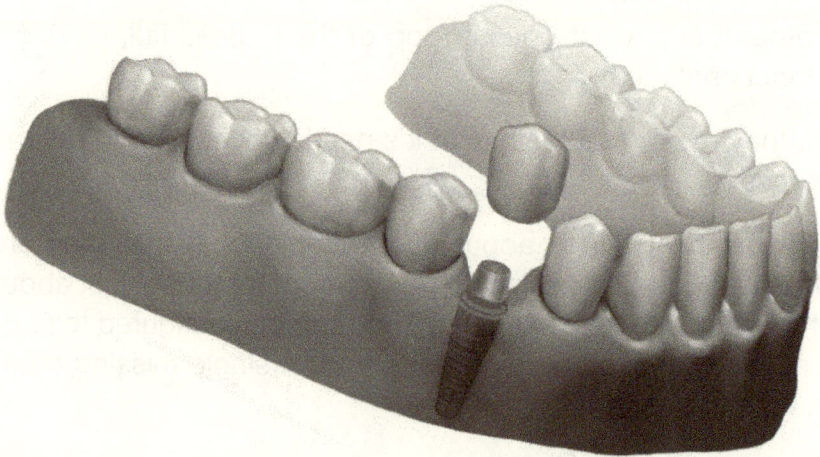

One way of transforming a titanium screw into something that looks just like a natural tooth is with a custom-made crown. The crown is attached to an abutment—a cap-like structure, also made of titanium—that serves as a base for the crown. Once the crown is attached to the abutment, it looks and acts just like a natural tooth—except for the added benefit that it will never decay.

Dental Implant Next to a Real Tooth

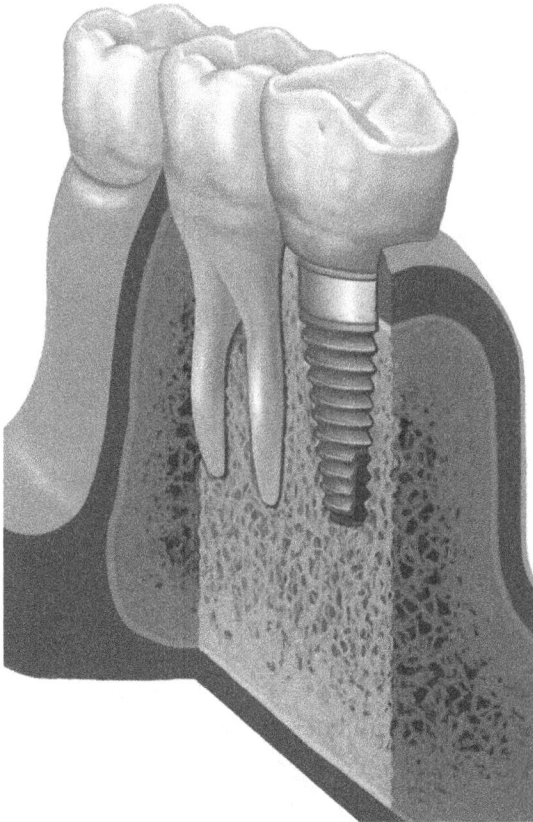

These crowns can be fixed or removable, and they can be attached to the implant either with cement (for a permanent implant) or a screw (for a removable one). Your dentist will work with you to determine exactly what options will work best for you.

Implants can also be used to support traditional dentures, improving in several ways on dentures that are held in place with adhesive. First, the implant itself will stop any bone loss from the area where the tooth has been lost, which will preserve the natural shape of your jaw.

Dentures Stabilized

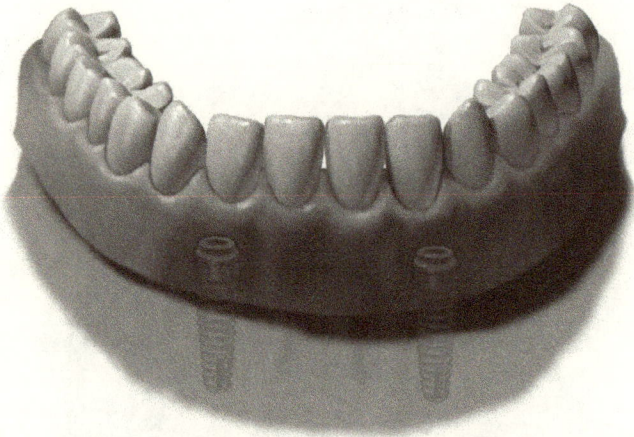

Dentures Supported

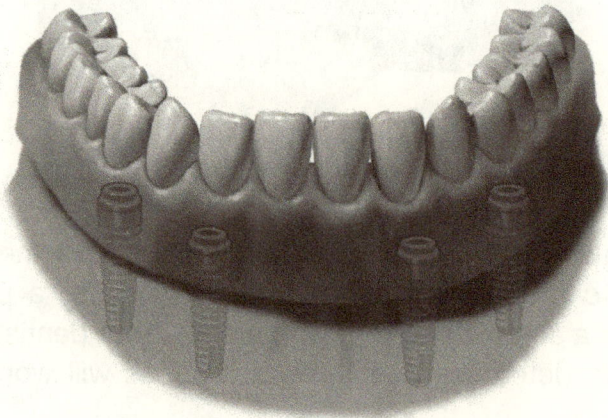

And finally, a dental implant provides a much more secure fit than denture adhesives, giving you a stronger bite, a more natural-looking smile, and the confidence you may be missing with dentures that slip and slide around in your mouth.

Basically, whatever your dental issues are, implants can likely help to provide the best, most modern, and most effective solution available.

Watch a free video on how to stop bone loss at **www.yourmissingteetharekillingyou.com**.

But Why Do We Still Lose Teeth?

To borrow an often-used phrase, "If we can put a man on the moon, why can't we prevent tooth loss entirely?" With all the advanced technology out there, with all the diseases that have been cured, it is pretty amazing that one-third of Americans over age sixty-five are missing not just some but all of their teeth.

You're in good company for a good reason. For many of us, our teeth just haven't evolved to the point where they can keep up with the rest of our bodies.

Luckily, science has evolved—and thanks to dental implants, we can continue to live with something almost exactly like our natural teeth that will last for the rest of our lives.

This is almost as good as putting a man on the moon.

Both Fred and Herman would certainly agree with that statement. These two stories are both very close to my heart. The first one is in the form of a letter I received from a former patient Fred. Fred has since passed away, so you can see why it's so special to me.

Herman is like a surrogate father to me. He and I have become close friends through the years. When I present seminars, he will speak to the audience about his experience with dental implants. He is so happy that we were able to throw his dentures in the trash!

Freddie's Story

"Fifteen years of misery due to receding gums and about seven sets of lower dentures, of which none fit well enough for me to eat what I wanted, but to eat what I could with the teeth I had to please my gums. Fixodent was with me everywhere so I could eat something that was on the menu. Because of the teeth and gums, I had to glue my teeth in every meal, every day (365 days a year).

"I went to several dentists, all telling me that I was not a candidate for implants, so I gave up on the idea for a long time.

"My wife and I moved to Florida in 1998, still with the same old trouble with my teeth. One day I was sitting at the dinner table looking at the paper and saw an ad on implants. I told my wife I was going to see this man and see if he could do anything for me. My wife said, 'You might as well save your time; you've been down that road before.' I decided to go see him anyway.

"I went to see him on January 11, 2006. They x-rayed my lower jaw (where my gums were supposed to be). The doctor looked at the x-ray and told me that he could put in implants and make me teeth that would do the job. My wife didn't want me to have this done because of my bad health. Also, a friend who had started a similar process up in Ohio told me it was so terrible. She begged me not to have it done.

"Even with all my bad health and the discouragement, I made up my mind I was going to have it done.

"When the implants were put in, I had very little pain afterward. I told the doctor that I would like for him to make it look like I had some lower teeth, because before when I ate a sandwich my nose would touch the sandwich bun before I could get it bit off. Now it is like a dream come true. I can bite the sandwich. Also, I can eat out when I want to. I eat chocolate-covered raisins, peanuts, and pecan pie, which I couldn't even think of eating before. So you know that I am a happy man with my teeth. Sure, I have to go back for adjustments sometimes, but I can do that gladly after all the problems I had.

"P.S. When we used to eat out with my best friend and his wife (they were best man and bridesmaid at our wedding), he always said that while he was eating his food, I was 'worrying mine to death.' Now I can finish my food before him."

* * *

Herman's Story

"I had false teeth that I despised. I wore them in my pocket more than I did in my mouth. They didn't fit well, and they were extremely uncomfortable, and when I talked they had a tendency to just fall out. That was a terrible experience, so I used my hands to hide my mouth a lot.

"I couldn't eat a lot of things. I had to eat very soft things. It didn't really affect my health a lot, but it certainly affected my eating. It was even hard to eat hamburgers or steak or anything else along those lines. So I kind of lived on soup and mashed potatoes.

"It was hard to face people. I had to be careful because I was afraid my teeth were going to fall out when I talked, so I always looked away from people. So people didn't think I was very friendly.

"I've had my implants a long time—over ten years. I had been looking for dental implants for a number of years, but people kept saying they weren't ready yet. Then I met a friend who… well, his teeth were really looking nice, so I asked who did it. He told me about his dentist, and I went in, and we discussed it, and I said, 'let's go.' I was ready for implants, and it sounded like he knew what he was talking about, so I said okay.

"That was ten years ago probably, and they're still in great shape. In some respects they're better than regular teeth—you don't get cavities. But the best part about it was that from the very first day, I took my false teeth and threw them away. I then got my temporary teeth put in. It was a great feeling. I thought, 'oh boy, I can now smile and not be ashamed, and when I go out to eat I won't have to hide myself behind a newspaper or a menu.'

"I could have stopped with the temporary teeth and never even gotten the implants. They were that much better. Immediately, food started tasting better. I could eat almost everything I wanted. It was a real plus to be able to immediately change my eating habits and my whole outlook on life.

"My thinking is that all we have is our health, and our health starts with our mouth. What we eat affects our health, and if our teeth aren't good and you can't eat right, you're not going to live much longer.

"Today, I'm eating better and living better and am more self-confident. I'm friendlier, and being friendlier, you accumulate more friends.

"So if you're thinking about implants at all, my advice is this. Don't hesitate, just have it done. You'll never, never be sorry."

* * *

CHAPTER 6

ARE YOU A CANDIDATE FOR DENTAL IMPLANTS?

I was hesitant because I thought it was going to be painful. But actually I didn t really feel any pain at all! I couldn t believe I didn t! I had four implants put in.

Don

I've provided a great deal of information in this book. You may be asking yourself the question, "Am I a candidate for dental implants?"

Perhaps for some reason you're thinking implants won't work for you. You may think that your situation is unique and you're the one for whom implants just won't work. Maybe you're worried that you'll just have to stick with your uncomfortable dentures forever and give up your dreams of having a natural-looking smile ever again.

In the vast majority of cases, not only do dental implants work, but they work beautifully. By this I mean they work for all kinds of patients with all kinds of problems. Modern dental implants are made in such a wide variety of sizes and types that they can accommodate nearly every situation.

How Healthy Do You Need to Be?

In order to be a candidate for dental implants, you need to be in generally good health. But the concept of generally good health is a lot less restrictive than it might sound, especially if you're a senior. Those normal aches and pains, and some of the common illnesses that come with getting older, should *not* prevent you from getting implants.

In fact, your age is absolutely not a factor when determining whether or not you are a good candidate for implants. It simply does not matter how old you are.

Why? Because implants and implant procedures have been designed specifically with older people in mind. Seniors make up the largest group of people who suffer from tooth loss, so it makes sense that implant technology is designed with their specific needs in mind.

If you're worried you might be too old for dental implants, that is just not the case! In fact, there's a saying that if you're healthy enough to get to the dentist, you're healthy enough for dental implants. This means that if you're in good enough shape to make it to your dentist's office, it's highly likely that the dentist can come up with a solution that works for you.

That doesn't mean there are absolutely no restrictions. You must be committed to taking care of your implants. That means regular dental visits, twice-yearly cleanings, and a commitment to take care of any problems quickly, before they get out of control.

Special Cases

Most dentists will also tell you that you must have healthy gums and enough bone to hold the implant. Of course, if you don't have healthy gums right now, your dentist can work with you to get them healthy enough to support implants. And if you've suffered from extreme bone loss, there are a variety of bone-grafting procedures available to build bone back up so that your jaw can support implants.

To learn more about bone grafting visit

www.yourmissingteetharekillingyou.com.

Even if you have some of these problems, you may well be able to get implants after you clear up these issues, such as getting a bone graft.

Still, there are some patients for whom the implant process can be just a little bit trickier. You might have read that smokers do not make good implant candidates, but if you discuss this with your dentist, chances are you can work out a plan to deal with it. It might even provide you with a little incentive to quit smoking!

Patients who have had radiation therapy to their head or neck area must be evaluated individually to see if implants will work for them.

Generally, people who suffer from chronic, uncontrolled diabetes or heart disease may not be candidates for dental implants. Again, you will have to consult with your physician and your dentist, as every situation is unique. This issue here is the level of control (or lack thereof) of the disease (e.g., uncontrolled diabetes). If you are seeing a doctor and getting treatment, there is always a good chance that your condition will improve and no longer be "uncontrolled."

If that happens, once you are healthy enough to get to the dentist's office and sit in the chair for a procedure, chances are your dentist can devise a plan to make dental implants a part of your new, healthier life.

The good news with all of this is that if you choose a board-certified implant dentist, he or she will do everything possible to find a way to make implants work for you. A thorough evaluation of your dental and overall health will be performed before any implant procedure begins.

Since the vast majority of patients can receive implants in some capacity, simply by disclosing your complete and total health history to your dentist, you enable him or her to work with you to design the treatment plan that will work for you. No two people are exactly alike, and no two implant-treatment plans are either.

The Good News

This means that for the majority of people reading this book, there is no question that dental implants will work for you. The success rate of dental implants is 98 to 100 percent, making them the most successful dental procedure available today.

So the only real question left is whether or not you believe you can benefit from them. And in almost every case, you can—and you will!

It's as simple as asking yourself such questions as the following:

Are dentures affecting your quality of life?

Do you find yourself missing the days when you could eat a wide variety of foods?

Have you lost your desire to eat, or even lost weight you didn't want to lose since you started wearing dentures?

Is the shape of your face changing?

Are you reluctant to talk or smile because your dentures cause embarrassment?

Are your dentures ever uncomfortable or even painful?

Do your dentures make you feel old?

Do you wish there was a better way?

If you answer yes to any of these questions, you will be amazed at the changes dental implants will make in your life. If you have a desire to enjoy family, food, friends, and an optimum quality of life for as long as possible—and as fully as possible—dental implants may be the miracle you are waiting for.

Should I Spend the Money?

Dental implants are an investment. You need to ask yourself a question: "Is it worth it to be able to chew anything I want, with confidence, and have the quality of life I deserve?" If you are in an assisted-living facility, a highlight of your day is going to the dining room and having a good meal, with no worries of "*I can t chew*" and being able to really *enjoy* your meal and your *friends!*

In your twilight years, isn't this *what really matters?* So make the investment in your health and your smile. Remember you are worth it!

A Word about Cost

An implant investment can range from nine hundred dollars to nineteen thousand dollars for the upper or lower jaw. Dental insurance plans will often pay a portion of the cost of the replacement teeth that attach to implants, and some medical insurance plans will cover part of the surgical treatment.

However, implants can actually be cost-effective when you consider the fact that your days of replacing dentures (that usually don't fit) will be over. And then consider the savings that result in enjoying improved overall health. Healthy people save a great deal of money in medical costs.

Additionally, you cannot place a price on how it feels to have your life back—to be able to work if you want to, travel, see friends, eat whatever you want (whenever you want and wherever you want!), and live an active, healthy life for many years to come.

Maybe that's why, in a survey of 350 patients who had dental-implant treatment, 97.6 percent felt it was well worth the investment and would absolutely do it all over again. And most say they would have done it sooner!

You deserve to feel like they do. You deserve to live every moment to the fullest and never worry about your teeth, beyond keeping them clean and taking care of them, of course.

That's why many dentists offer third-party financing and other payment plans to help you afford the dental work you need. If you're worried about how you will be able to afford dental implants, don't simply dismiss it as something that's not for you. Talk with your dentist about your unique situation. Chances are he or she will be able to work out a plan for you.

With regard to the cost of implants, I like the way Don puts it all in perspective—with a little humor thrown in.

Don's Story

"I grew up in a coal mining town, and my father was a coal miner. I had thirty-five cavities before I was in my twenties, and then even more later on in my life, so I knew I would eventually need some pulled. Later I had all of my back molars removed on one side because I would always chew on only one side of my mouth.

"At one point I had saved up enough money to buy a BMW. It was either the BMW or the dental work. So now I tell people I have a BMW in my mouth. (My little joke!)

"I wasn't able to chew well before implants. For instance, I'd have to cut up an apple to eat it. Now I can eat the entire apple whole if I want, and pretty much eat anything else I want.

"I do try to be careful with really hard foods, because I don't want to crack the implant, but that is just basic care, I would think. That's common sense.

"Before dental implants, my self-esteem about my smile was definitely affected. I would cover my mouth with my hand, and I tried not to smile too much because I did not like the way I looked.

"My dentist back in Illinois started talking about dental implants years ago, but at the time I was not in a position to afford them.

"I always knew I would need something done, but I also knew I was never going to get dentures. Just the thought of putting them in and out, and cleaning them every day, sounded like such a hassle.

"Once I came down to Florida, I started seeing the same dentist's print ads, and I finally decided one day that I was going to make an appointment for a consultation!

"He thoroughly explained the details of the procedure and how it would really make a positive impact on my life. I was hesitant because I thought it was going to be painful. But actually I didn't really feel any pain at all! I couldn't believe I didn't! I had four implants put in.

"Dental implants have really changed my self-esteem, as I can give my big BMW smile now! I can eat whatever I want, and I know that those teeth are fixed in there, and I don't have to worry about them coming out.

"For anyone who is looking to get dental implants, I would say that the procedure is worth it. It can make such a huge impact on your life, on your self-confidence, and on your health. I still won't eat a steak, because I just don't eat steak, but knowing that I can eat anything I want is a huge benefit."

★ ★ ★

CHAPTER 7

HOW TO CHOOSE AN IMPLANT DENTIST

> *I hated eating in front of people, because I didn t know if my partial denture would become loose. When this happened, I would have to excuse myself and go to the restroom to put my teeth back in place.*
>
> *Terry*

Once you decide to improve your smile and your life with dental implants, you still have one more major decision to make. Who are you going to trust with the very important job of performing your implant procedure? While the success rate of dental implants is remarkably high, it is still a very complex job. Therefore, it's extremely important that you choose a qualified dental professional to perform the implant procedures. Every major dental school in America offers instruction in dental implants. This proves implants have become the industry standard when it comes to treating tooth loss, and it means a qualified implant dentist should not be terribly difficult to find in your area.

That's why, while any licensed dentist is allowed by law to provide dental implants, *you* need to choose the right person to restore *your* smile.

My suggestion is to interview the implant dentist and find out the following:

- How many implants has he placed in his career?
- Does he do all the procedures, or will he be sending you all over town to multiple dentists (which for most people is an inconvenience)?
- Does he do them routinely?
- Does he have any patients whom you could talk to, and has he placed implants for them?
- Does he have board-certification status? How much training has he had, and does he keep up with all the new cutting-edge technology that helps implant dentistry make tremendous strides and assure that the procedure is more predictable and successful?

Who Performs Dental Implant Surgery?

Dental professionals in several categories perform implant surgery.

Dentists

Many dentists are qualified and experienced with dental implants. The term DDS, which is the degree most dentists earn in dental school, actually means doctor of dental surgery. And the DMD degree means doctor of dental medicine. As all dentists must earn a college degree and complete four years of dental school, they are very highly trained. They are also required to hold a license to practice in the state where they work, so they must meet and maintain certain standards in order to be allowed to practice.

To be certified in any of the following dental specialties, a dentist needs to complete additional years of training.

GENERAL DENTISTS

Your dentist may have taken extended training, like yearlong implant courses given by implant training institutes, for example, the Misch Implant Institute or the AAID (American Academy of Implant Dentistry) MaxiCourse. If your dentist is trained properly, he can perform all phases of implant dentistry and doesn't need to send you to other dentists. He also can achieve board certification credentials, which sets him apart from other general dentists and provides information on the level of advance training he has (visit WWW.ABOI.ORG and WWW.ICOI.ORG)

Your dentist may also refer you to one of the following dental specialists if your teeth, gums, bite, or supporting bone structure needs to be evaluated more specifically. Since the condition of any of those can affect the way implants will work for you, before you start, you may need to be treated for conditions that might get in the way of a successful implant treatment.

Oral and/or Maxillofacial Surgeons

Oral surgeons specialize in treating mouth and jaw problems where surgery is required. In situations where your teeth are badly damaged, or some of them are missing, your dentist may refer you to an oral surgeon.

Prosthodontists

Prosthodontic dentists concentrate on replacing or saving teeth by repairing, restoring, or replacing them. They also deal with the structures in the mouth and jaw that relate to teeth. Any dentist who has graduated from an accredited dental school is allowed to practice prosthodontics. A three-year, post-doctoral training program is also available, as is a board certification by the American Board of Prosthodontics, which a dentist needs to pass a four-part examination to obtain. Board-certified prosthodontists must be recertified every eight years to keep up with changes in technology.

Periodontists

A periodontist is a dentist who specializes in gum disease; periodontists diagnose it, help prevent it, and treat it. If you have serious gum problems, you may need to see a periodontist to have those issues addressed before you can get dental implants, and your periodontist may perform implant procedures. Periodontists must complete three additional years of training after dental school.

Any one of these dentists might be the right person to provide you with dental implants. Now, the question is, how do you go about finding the professional who is right for you?

Step 1: Get Names

It's important that you know something about your implant doctor before the surgery begins. You'll most likely want to look into a few candidates in your area to help you find the one who is the best fit for you.

The best place to start is by consulting with your current dentist, provided you have one you trust. After all, your dentist knows your mouth and your teeth better than anyone else and has at least some idea of what it will take to fit you with dental implants.

He or she may have training in this area and be able to do the implants, or, if you need a specialist, he or she may refer you to a trusted colleague he knows.

Of course, you can also ask family, friends, coworkers, and colleagues, especially if any of them have had, or know someone who has had, implant surgery. If you know someone with an amazing smile that didn't come entirely from nature, find out where it did come from! It could lead you to an implant dentist worth getting to know.

If you have absolutely no connections to any implant dentists, you may learn about someone who practices in your area from an ad on TV, on the radio, in a magazine or newspaper, or a flyer in your mailbox. There's nothing wrong with finding your implant doctor through an advertisement. After all, those ads are designed to let patients just like you know about the doctor who is doing the advertising. Just remember that the information in an advertisement is there to get you to come to the office. Before deciding to let anyone create your new smile, you should learn all you can about any dentist. In other words, you need to do your homework.

Step 2: Research

Simply getting an implant dentist's name or a recommendation from someone you know is only the beginning. Even if your dentist recommends a specialist to you, it's always a good idea to do some investigating on your own, if possible, before you set up an appointment for a consultation.

Many dentists have websites where you can find out where they went to school, what their training is, how many years they've been in practice, and their experience with implants.

If they don't have a website, request the information from them. You don't need to be embarrassed or feel like you're being pushy or demanding. This is your smile we're talking about! And when choosing the person who is going to be responsible for your new smile, experience is key. The more training and experience your dentist has had, the better it will be for you.

Ideally, you want to find a dentist who has been trained or certified by at least one of these groups that specialize in implants:

- American Board of Oral Implantology/Implant Dentistry (ABOI/ID)
- American Academy of Periodontists (AAP)
- American Academy of Implant Dentistry (AAID)
- International Congress of Oral Implantologists (ICOI)

- Misch International Implant Institute (MIII)
- American College of Prosthodontists (ACP)
- American Academy of Implant Prosthodontics (AAIP)

Ask to see before-and-after pictures of the dentist's implant patients. This will give you an idea of the number and types of patients the dentist has worked with and the type of work he or she does. And make sure these are actual photos of actual patients, not general before-and-after pictures you might see on the Internet. It helps if the dentist can share stories of who these people are and how their procedures went.

Make sure the dentist is up-to-date on the latest technology. Ask how the dentist's practice will address your comfort and ease any anxieties you might have while you're undergoing treatment. Ask what sort of sedation they use and what extra touches— video, music, massage chairs—they have in the office. Finally, while implants are safe and have the highest success rate in dentistry today, find out how the dentist would handle an emergency, especially one that takes place after hours.

I can't stress enough that you shouldn't be embarrassed about asking a lot of questions. Dental implants can change your life. You have every right to find the right professional.

Here are some questions you should be sure to ask your implant dentist before going forward with treatment:

1. How long have you been in practice?
2. How many implant procedures have you done?
3. When was the last time you did an implant procedure?
4. Where did you receive your training?
5. May I speak with some of your former patients?
6. May I see before-and-after photos?
7. What is your success rate?
8. How will you deal with my discomfort during and after the procedure?

9. Will you also be handling my crowns, or will another dentist need to do it?
10. Will I have to leave your office or spend any time in public without teeth?

If you are uncomfortable with an implant doctor's answers to any of these questions, schedule an appointment with someone else. Meet with as many doctors as you need to feel secure and comfortable. Remember, the more you know about your potential implant dentist before your treatment, the more you increase your chances of having the best experience—and the best outcome—possible.

When one of my patients, Terry, was thinking about getting implants, he thought it was going to be terribly painful. Read how Terry describes his experience getting implants.

Terry's Story

"I am sixty-four years old and in the process of having three implants done, which are replacing a partial I had for almost thirty years.

"I hated eating in front of people, because I didn't know if my partial would become loose. When this happened, I would have to excuse myself and go to the restroom to put my teeth back in place. I had to be careful what I ordered to eat. I also had to worry about food getting behind the wire of my partial and underneath my partial.

"The implant process wasn't anything like I expected it to be. I thought it would be painful, but it wasn't very painful at all. I didn't even need prescription painkillers but simply took Tylenol for the discomfort. I put ice on the area, so the swelling was very little. Each implant is a process, but for each one the recovery period was just two or three days.

"As I said before, getting implants has been a process. I had two at one time, then had the third. The anchors had to go in first, and there is a process of about ten weeks of healing for each implant. I kept getting filled so I was never without teeth.

"I have temporary teeth in now, and I can already eat with ease, just with the temporary teeth. The next time I go back I will have an impression made for my permanent teeth. When they are completed, the temporary teeth will be removed, and the permanent teeth will be connected to the implants. I am so looking forward to what they will look like. I am excited about getting my permanent teeth in. It is going to be great!

"If you're even thinking about it, my advice is don't do like I did and put off getting implants. Get it done as soon as possible. It is so much better to be able to smile without being self-conscious. Plus, you don't have to worry about dentures embarrassing you when you are eating.

"My implants are on the bottom, and I have a complete upper denture. My dream is to one day have the upper dentures replaced with implants."

* * *

CHAPTER 8

YOUR FIRST OFFICE VISIT

In my estimation, you cannot put a price on good health. Like I said, without it you have nothing.

Dave

Planning your implant procedures is kind of like remodeling a room in your house. Before anything actually happens, your dentist will examine your mouth and your teeth to get a complete picture of where you are, where you want to go, and the best way to help you get there.

Prior to scheduling your implant surgery, you will have a consultation with your dentist that will help you decide on the best course of treatment. The consultation is where all the planning for your future new teeth takes place, so it is a very important step. You and your dentist will determine everything from what will work for you to what your new smile will actually look like. And, most importantly, you will know exactly what to expect from your upcoming implant procedure.

The Implant Consultation

A consultation appointment can be an exciting time, especially if you get the opportunity to see yourself with a beautiful new smile. Remember, the point of the consultation is to help you choose the implant doctor who is right for you. Visit several implant doctors until you find the one you feel totally comfortable with.

You want to feel confident about both your implant dentist and the course of treatment he or she recommends for you.

It's advisable to compare as many candidates as possible—even if that means having multiple consultations—to help you decide on the one who is right for you. Remember, you only have one smile, so you deserve the best.

Once You ve Decided

So you've selected your implant dentist and are ready to move forward. Congratulations! Soon you will be facing the world with a beautiful new smile. But before you reach that point, your dentist will schedule a clinical evaluation to come up with a comprehensive plan to make sure that your new smile is strong and healthy and will last as long as you do.

Because dental implants can be a complex procedure, there are several steps involved in a clinical-evaluation appointment. Be sure to set aside well over an hour to spend with your implant doctor and staff so that he or she can completely address all of your needs.

Most or all of the following steps will be included in your diagnostic evaluation.

Medical History

Your implant doctor needs to have a clear picture of both your physical health and your dental health to design the right implant plan for you. If you have access to your comprehensive medical and/or dental records, be sure to bring them in for your implant doctor to look at. They will tell more about you than you might even know about yourself. If not, your implant doctor may ask for a list of your current medical and dental providers.

Your implant doctor will ask you about any and all medications you are currently taking, including any over-the-counter drugs. Don't be embarrassed to tell the truth. This is strictly for your safety, as some drugs interact badly with other drugs, and others can affect bleeding and healing. You should also inform your implant dentist if you suffer from any medical conditions, like heart disease or diabetes.

Oral Exam

Every mouth is different, and your implant doctor needs to have a full and complete understanding of your unique situation. So a complete oral exam is a major and necessary part of the clinical-evaluation process. Your tongue and the soft tissues of your mouth will be checked for oral cancer, and your implant doctor will also check the lymph nodes in your neck. The health of your gums will be evaluated. Your remaining teeth will be checked for decay and periodontal disease as well as mobility, meaning how firmly they are secured in your jaw.

Your implant doctor will check the bone in the area where your teeth are missing, or where they will eventually be extracted, to determine how much remains and the quality of what is there. If the bone in these areas is not thick enough to support an implant, additional procedures such as bone grafting may be necessary.

Finally, your doctor will study your facial symmetry to see if your jaws and other facial features are properly aligned or if other procedures are needed to bring them back into alignment.

X-Rays

X-rays will give your implant doctor a clearer picture of what's going on inside your mouth. They help determine whether you have enough bone in specific areas, such as above the nerve in your lower jaw (for lower implants) and below your sinus cavity on your upper jaw (for upper implants in the back of the jaw). X-rays will also give your implant dentist a better idea of how dense your bone is. While there is no way to know your exact bone density until implant surgery is actually performed, x-rays will show any problem areas.

At this point, many implant dentists also like to do a panoramic x-ray that gives the dentist a sort of all-around view of your mouth and teeth. CT scans or CAT scans are another diagnostic tool used in treatment planning your case. It's all designed to give your implant doctor the best possible picture of your mouth.

Impressions

If you had braces when you were a child, you may have had impressions taken before. Dentists take impressions by having you bite down into a tray filled with a putty-like substance, which is used to create an exact model of your jaws, teeth, and gums that gives your implant doctor a physical representation of how your teeth are shaped and how they come together. It can be used to help your doctor design your new teeth or to plan exactly where implants will go for the most successful and lifelike restoration of your smile.

Photographs

This step is basically self-explanatory. Your implant doctor, or perhaps an assistant, will take a series of photos of your face and your smile. These will also be used to design your replacement teeth, as well as to document what you looked like before you received your new smile.

Choosing New Teeth

Together with your implant doctor, you will decide on the shade and color of crowns that will be standing in for your old teeth. If you will be mixing these new teeth with natural teeth, you obviously want the color to match perfectly so that the look is seamless. If you will be replacing all of your teeth, the doctor and his staff will help you choose the color that looks the best *and* is the most natural.

The Plan

By the conclusion of your diagnostic evaluation, your implant dentist should be ready to devise a plan to create the beautiful new smile you want and deserve.

He or she will discuss the reconstruction options that will work best for you, the number of implants you will need, and any special needs you might have, like additional bone reconstruction, to make your implant surgery a success.

You will also discuss the cost of your treatment and any insurance or payment options that might be available to you. And you might go so far as to schedule your implant surgery or any other procedure that needs to be done beforehand.

You will, of course, be informed of the different types of anesthesia that will work in your case, how to prepare for your surgery, and what to do during your recovery, including what to do about pain, what you can eat and when, when you can resume normal activity, and how to care for your mouth and replacement teeth after surgery.

Your implant doctor will explain how long your treatment will take and whether or not you will have to go without teeth for any period of time. Please understand that leaving your implant dentist's office without teeth is usually *not* necessary! If your implant doctor tells you that this cannot be helped, ask why. If it has more to do with his or her capabilities than it does with your case, you may want to look into another implant dentist who can give you a new smile without causing you undue embarrassment.

Erasing Fears

As your appointment winds down, you will be able to share any questions or concerns you might have with your implant doctor, so you can be sure you understand what is going on and are totally comfortable with your upcoming procedure. Don't be afraid to ask any questions you might have. Your implant doctor should be used to them, and he or she should be able to answer them in a way that will ease your fears.

The implant process might sound complex and scary, but it really isn't. It is actually a fairly simple outpatient surgery with an extremely high success rate. All this preparation is necessary to insure that your implant surgery results in a beautiful smile that will last you for the rest of your life.

So don't be intimidated by everything that goes on during your pre-implant visit. When your implant surgery goes smoothly, when you wake up with a mouth full of beautiful new teeth, you will understand how completely life changing this type of surgery can be. I promise you, it's all worth it.

In the next chapter, I'll explain more about the actual implant treatment, but first let Dave and Margaret tell you their experiences with implants.

Dave's Story

"I've had my implants for a little over two years. I just turned sixty-four, and I was sixty-one when I got them. I had had my teeth taken out and dentures put in at a clinic up in South Carolina, and they did an absolutely lousy job. They didn't do everything that they were supposed to. The dentures did not fit properly, and I had an impacted wisdom tooth that they were supposed to remove and didn't. It was just a big mess.

"I had difficulty eating some things, like corn on the cob and steaks and things of that nature. The dentures had a tendency to want to slip out. My wife and I like to take cruises, and when you're sitting at a table with six other couples, and you go to bite into something, and your dentures slip out, it's rather embarrassing.

"I felt restricted, like I had to be careful. I wound up getting a cloth denture adhesive that I would use to help hold the dentures in place. It helped a little, but eventually the adhesive would wear off before the end of the day, and I wound up having to replace it a couple times a day, and you're not supposed to do that. I had to break the rules just to keep my teeth in my mouth.

"At first, I just wanted to get new dentures. But then I decided to go with implants, and I'm very glad that I did.

"The process was virtually painless. My gums, which had been messed up from having my teeth removed at the clinic, were straightened, and I had the impacted wisdom tooth removed. I had a little bit of discomfort the following day, but I only had to take a little pain medicine. As far as pain, no. There was no real pain at all.

"I woke up with new teeth. They were only temporary, but I did not walk out of that office without teeth in my mouth. I was totally amazed. I really was. The whole procedure took six or seven months total before I got my permanent dentures, but even the temporary ones were a big, big improvement over what I had.

"Within a couple of days, until my gums healed, I was on a soft diet, so I didn't rip out any of the sutures or anything. I'd say in less than a week's time I was back to eating regular food without any problems whatsoever—real food, like I ate when I had regular teeth. It has made a big difference. I have no fear of eating anything. I can eat steak and corn on the cob, anything like that, and I do not have the fear of my dentures slipping out and embarrassing me anymore. I don't have to worry about packing the denture adhesive when I take a cruise with my wife. They're just a part of me now. They look and feel natural.

"If you can't eat and chew properly, you don't have good health. If you don't have good health, you don't have anything at all. Being able to eat anything that I want, when I want, and knowing that it's doing me good and that my health's good, what it cost me to have the work done was well worth it. In my estimation, you cannot put a price on good health. Like I said, without it you have nothing."

* * *

Margaret's Story

"I've had my implants for around ten years, and I love them. I'm a professional person, and for that reason my appearance is very important to me. I was missing lower teeth, and it affected my appearance and my self-confidence.

"I had a partial plate for a time, but it was extremely uncomfortable. Having a full set of lower dentures was not feasible for me because I didn't have enough bone to hold in a denture.

"The work that I had done was somewhat different from most others who get implants. I first needed to have bone and skin built up. I have to say, that part was painful and unpleasant. However, the outcome was worth it all!

"Today, all these years later, I'm very happy with my teeth and also my improved appearance. I would absolutely recommend implants to anyone who is considering taking that step."

* * *

CHAPTER 9

YOUR IMPLANT TREATMENT

I was determined I would never have teeth like stars the kind that came out at night. I had no desire to be taking my teeth in and out and in and out every day for the rest of my life.

Patti

Now It s Your Turn

Finally, after all the planning and questioning and preparation, the big moment has arrived. It's time for your implant surgery— time to start your new life with your new, improved smile. But before you start that new life, you're probably wondering just what to expect from your implant treatment (or treatments). Maybe you're even feeling a little nervous or frightened.

When you're planning your treatment, your implant dentist will tell you in detail exactly what is going to happen every step of the way. This chapter will provide a sense of how implant treatments are done and the steps involved in creating your new smile.

There are two basic types of dental-implant procedures. The standard procedure is performed over a period of three to six months, depending on how long it takes the implant, or implants, to osseointegrate, or fuse with the jawbone. In other cases, your implant doctor may perform a one-stage surgical procedure in which a second implant surgery is not necessary.

Which type of procedure is used depends on a variety of factors, including your implant doctor's specialties, the extent of the restoration you need done, the type of implants you'll be receiving, and the type of temporary prosthetic you will be using during the healing process.

I'll describe both types of procedures in detail here.

The Standard Implant Procedure

A standard implant procedure involves three separate stages:

1. Preparing the jaw and placing the implants

2. Uncovering the implants and attaching temporary crowns

3. Attaching permanent crowns, which is also called "loading" the implants

During the first stage, you will either be given a sedative or given local or general anesthesia, depending on your implant doctor and the extent of the surgery required. This is to make sure you won't feel any pain or discomfort during the procedure. You'll want to ask if you will need a driver to take you home after your appointment. You cannot drive for a period of time after receiving conscious sedation, and driving while sedated is never a good idea! You'll also want to wear loose, comfortable clothing so that you can fully relax during your treatment.

Your surgery will take anywhere from one hour to several hours, depending on how much work is being done. In most cases, it is performed right in the dentist's chair. Your implant doctor will begin by removing any teeth that are going to be replaced due to disease or damage. Once the area has been cleared for your new teeth, your implant doctor will make tiny incisions in your gums wherever an implant is going to be inserted. Small holes will be prepared in your jawbone, and titanium implants will be surgically placed inside and covered with protective tops called cover screws. After the implants are in place, your gums will be sutured closed and left to heal while the implants fuse with your bone.A temporary denture will be inserted so you will NEVER LEAVE THE OFFICE WITHOUT TEETH!

After surgery, ice will be used to reduce swelling in your jaw. Your gums will likely still be numb when you leave the office. Patients are usually ready to go home about half an hour after surgery. When the numbness wears off, you may feel some discomfort, so be sure to ask your implant dentist about your options for pain relief. You'll also be given a prescription for some kind of antibiotic to prevent infection.

You will probably want to rest when you get home, and you may need to stay off your feet for a day or two. Your implant doctor will give you specific instructions to help you take care of your mouth to make sure you heal properly. You will be advised on dealing with any bleeding that might take place, what you can eat and when, and how to keep your mouth clean while you are healing. If you experience any problems like fever, severe pain, an increase in swelling, or heavy bleeding, call your implant doctor right away. Remember, it's always better to be safe than sorry. Your implant doctor will want to know if you are having any problems.

After the initial surgery, you will need to wait three to six months while your implants are osseointegrated, or fused with your natural bone. In the meantime, you will be provided with some sort of temporary prosthesis—either a partial denture that can be removed or a semi-permanent bridge that is glued in temprorary and doesn't come out

The second stage of the standard implant procedure takes place three to six months later, after your implants have fused to your jawbone and essentially become a part of you. You'll go back to your implant dentist and will be given a local anesthetic to numb the area. Your dentist will then uncover your implants. He or she will then remove the cover screws and attach abutments, which will hold both the temporary and permanent crowns in place. The incisions will be sutured, and temporary crowns, bridges, or dentures may be attached to the abutments, or you may be given a soft denture to wear while you heal.

As this is also a surgical procedure, you may again experience some discomfort as the anesthetic wears off, although most patients don't report feeling much pain. Just like last time, your implant dentist will advise you on how to manage any pain you might have, how to help your mouth heal, how to keep your mouth clean, and what you can eat and how soon. Recovery will be much faster and simpler than recovery from the first stage, but you should still be sure to follow your implant doctor's instructions closely to make sure everything heals properly for the next stage.

The Really Exciting Part

The final stage—called the restoration phase—takes place a few weeks later. Your implant dentist will take impressions of your jaw, including your abutments, to help make the permanent crowns, bridges, or dentures that will soon be your new, permanent teeth. You will probably have had impressions taken before your implant procedure began, so you will know what to expect. If you've forgotten, this means that you bite down in a tray of a putty-like substance, and the impression left indicates exactly where your implants are located in your jawbone.

The impression will be sent to a lab, where a model will be made of the inside of your mouth. That model will be used to create replacement teeth that will look and feel just like natural teeth and give you the dazzling new smile—and all the extras that come with it—that you've been waiting for!

When your new teeth are ready, you'll go back to your implant dentist for the big moment—what is called "loading" the implants, which basically means attaching your new, permanent teeth to the abutments. Your implant doctor will make sure your new teeth blend in and fit perfectly with your natural teeth.

And you'll be ready for a lifetime of more comfortable eating, talking, smiling and most importantly giving you back your SELF ESTEEM.

The One-Stage Implant Procedure

In some cases, the surgical aspect of your implant procedure can be taken care of in a single visit, so you will only need to be anesthetized (and recover) once. This is called a one-stage surgical procedure.

There are two major differences between a one-stage procedure and a standard procedure. The first is that in a one-stage procedure, the implants and abutments are placed in your mouth at the same time rather than during two separate surgeries. To make sure your gums don't grow back over the implants during healing, small caps called healing caps are placed over each implant.

The second major difference is that while osseointegration is taking place and your implants are fusing to your jawbone, you may not wear a temporary prosthesis, and if you do, it will likely be a denture that is loose and removable. For this reason, implant doctors tend to use the one-stage implant procedure in the back of the mouth where your teeth won't be seen, although there are other occasions, like replacement of a single tooth, when it is also the preferred method.

Other than the difference in prosthetics and the additional presence of healing caps, recovery after a one-stage implant procedure is generally similar to recovery from the first stage of a standard procedure. Your implant doctor will advise you of specifics regarding pain management, eating, cleaning, and healing, and it will still take months for your implants to fuse with your jawbone and become a permanent, nearly natural part of *you*.

Teeth in a Day   Immediately Loaded Implants

Imagine walking into your implant doctor's office and walking out with teeth.

Believe it or not, it is possible, with what dentists call immediately loaded implants. Thanks to recent advances in implant technology, many implant patients are now able to experience this instant and dramatic transformation.

The technique works best on patients who have enough bone remaining to immediately support the implant. It is an ideal choice for someone who needs to have a single tooth removed and wants an instant replacement. However, many implant dentists perform some version of the procedure, so be sure to ask yours if he or she performs the technique and if it will work for you. For many implant patients, immediately loaded implants are a very workable solution.

Of course, like any implant, immediately loaded implants still need several months of gentle care while osseointegration takes place, and there will also probably be a wait for permanent crowns or other tooth replacements. The primary advantage is that patients never, ever need to worry about facing the world without teeth again—even for a minute. And since that's why you're getting implants in the first place, there's nothing more exciting than getting that result in a single visit.

Of course, whatever method is ultimately best for you, the result will be the same. Within a few months, you will have beautiful, permanent teeth firmly rooted in your jaw. Any bone loss you are suffering will be stopped. You will be able to eat what you want, do what you want, and talk without embarrassment.

And of course, you'll be able to smile like you haven't smiled in years. And you'll be smiling that way for the rest of your life.

Patricia—see her story below—refers to her implants as giving her self-satisfaction. I like that statement.

And then we have Patti story. Hers was not a tooth problem, but a gum problem. No matter what the problem, she was bound and determined she would never be taking dentures in and out for the rest of her life. We helped make her dream come true! The teeth she has now never have to come out—ever!

Patricia's Story

"I currently have six dental implants. Five were put in back in 1996 and then another one just two years ago.

"Before the implants, I had a partial on the side. I didn't have any real problems with the partials, no difficulty chewing, because they made me a partial that was adequate to start. However, I got tired of taking them out, and I thought it would be wonderful to not have to remove those partials all the time.

"My husband had cancer, and during the radiation they had to replace all his teeth with bone rods. So he had just about all of his teeth removed, and he needed dentures. During the course of the conversation, the topic of implants came up. I had no real problems with my partials because they were well done, and implants were quite expensive, but I began to consider getting them.

"When I had them done, I was just under general anesthesia, and the dentist did all five at one time with absolutely no problem. It was a long procedure, but I've never had any problem with them. Everything just went perfectly.

"I had dreaded getting implants, afraid of going under anesthesia like with any surgery, but I've been very happy with my implants. I love my teeth; they mean a lot to me. When they were gone, it was like something was missing. Having the implants and permanent teeth again—it's self-satisfaction."

* * *

Patti's Story

"I'm seventy-three years old. I never had problems with my teeth, but I did have major problems with my gums. My gums were diseased and periodically had to be scraped. I knew sooner or later something would have to be done to correct the situation—it was just a matter of time. I was determined I would never have teeth like stars—the kind that came out at night. I had no desire to be taking my teeth in and out and in and out every day for the rest of my life.

"I learned about implants and watched a video, which explained the procedure and all that was involved. I never hesitated. I said, 'I'm going to do that.'

"I went home and talked with my husband. We both knew it was going to cost a lot of money. But he agreed with me that this was the best route to take.

"I was a great candidate for implants. I'm an active person and very healthy. I work as an instructor at the YMCA, where I've taught aerobics for thirty years.

"My implants were on the top only. Once the process began, it took almost a year to get it totally completed. Because of the 'twilight sleep' anesthetic, I was never uncomfortable during any of the office sessions. I was never in a great deal of discomfort afterward either. The pain level was handled only with Tylenol and ice packs—no prescription pain relievers. And I never missed a day of work.

"I still look back and think how amazing it all is. First of all, I was never without teeth. I think people considering implants need to know that. I always had temporary teeth throughout the process. And my new teeth are beautiful. I'm proud of them and know that it has helped my appearance a great deal.

I love my implants, and I d do it all over again in a heart-beat.

* * *

CHAPTER 10

LIVING WITH YOUR IMPLANTS

Now I can bite an apple. I eat all the foods I could years ago. It s been an improvement to my self-esteem, as well.

Grant

Best It s Ever Been!

The first thing you'll probably notice about living with dental implants is that it's almost exactly like life was years ago, when you had all of your natural teeth. After all, implants are designed to look, feel, and work just like the teeth you were born with because they actually become a part of your mouth.

Living with dental implants means you can eat whatever you want to without worrying. Bite into a crunchy apple—no more cutting it into little pieces. Enjoy some corn right off the cob. Munch down on a hero sandwich. Whatever you're hungry for, your teeth will most likely be ready to handle it!

But life with implants is about more than just eating. It's about getting out there and really living.

Really Living

It means you can talk with your friends and family without worrying if they can understand you or that your dentures might be making clicking noises. You can now laugh long and hard with your mouth wide-open, knowing your teeth won't slip. It's about exercising, traveling, working, socializing, and even getting romantic—and feeling totally and completely confident doing it. You'll be doing it all without having to wonder if your teeth will cause you any pain, discomfort, or embarrassment.

But the best part of living with your new implants is probably smiling at the people you love—and even people you don't know—with complete ease and comfort.

It's going to be an incredible feeling. And it's a feeling that's going to stay with you for the rest of your life.

Of course, eventually, after you've lived with your implants for a while, you'll start to think of them in basically the same way you used to think of your natural teeth. This means you'll probably reach a point where you'll live your life without thinking much about your implants at all.

A Fresh Start

Please understand, this doesn't mean that once all your implant procedures are behind you, your implants have osseointegrated, and your mouth has completely healed, you'll never have to think about your teeth again.

Look at it this way. Back when you had natural teeth, you might have had to think about them at least a couple of times a day. You had to brush them after eating to keep them clean. You had to floss them to keep your gums healthy. And you had to visit your dentist regularly to have your teeth professionally cleaned and to make sure your mouth stayed healthy and disease-free.

Then again, there's a change in that maybe you didn't exactly do all those things, even though you were supposed to. Not every-one does, after all. So maybe you were one of those people who didn't exactly take the best care of your natural teeth back when you had them.

Maybe that's part of the reason why you don't have those teeth anymore.

But however you lost your teeth in the first place, those days—just like the days when you didn't have teeth and had to get by with uncomfortable dentures—are now completely behind you. They're over. You have a new smile, a new you, and a new opportunity to do things differently.

Think of your new smile as a fresh start—the start of an exciting new life for you. And since you're starting a brand-new life any-way, now is an ideal time to adopt some new habits.

Develop Good Hygiene Habits

You want to keep your implants clean for the same reason you needed to keep your natural teeth clean: to make sure they last a lifetime. And the key to making sure teeth last a lifetime, whether they come from the man upstairs or the dentist across town, is preventing bone loss. Keep the bone around your implants healthy, and they will remain solidly secured in your jaw. And that's true whether or not that was the case with your natural teeth. Remember, your new implants are a fresh start.

You prevent bone loss by keeping your gums healthy. And your gums stay healthy when you keep your teeth, or in this case, your implants and prosthetic teeth, sparkling clean and free of plaque and tartar.

Since implants aren't exactly like natural teeth, the procedure for keeping them clean is a little different than what you might have done (or might not have done) to keep your natural teeth clean in the past. The specifics of how you will clean your particular implants will depend on the type of prosthetic teeth you have and whether they're crowns or dentures. But there are some general steps that you'll likely need to follow in some form or other.

Toothbrushes and More

Just like your mom told you when you were a kid, you should brush your implants—as well as any natural teeth you might have—after every meal. If you have a single implant with a crown that replaces a single tooth, either in one spot or in multiple places in your mouth, a standard toothbrush and fluoride tooth-paste (to keep your natural teeth healthy!) should be fine. Use standard, sonic, or rotary toothbrushes to clean the fronts, sides, and chewing surfaces of most types of implants.

But implants also present some special cleaning challenges. So there are special kinds of brushes that can be especially help-ful in keeping implants—and the areas around them—clean and plaque-free.

Splayed-bristle brushes have longer bristles on the sides, with shorter ones in the center. These longer bristles can wrap around and actually get under your prosthetic tooth, cleaning areas a normal toothbrush can't reach.

End-tufted brushes look like paintbrushes, but you don't need to be an artist to use them. These brushes have stiff bristles that work really well cleaning implants with bridges, especially when it comes to cleaning the insides of your teeth (on the tongue side of your mouth) up where they meet your gums. End-tufted brushes can even reach under a bridge to clean your abutments.

Interproximal brushes, which look like tiny Christmas trees, are very soft and flexible, so they're great for getting into tight spots and cleaning your abutments.

Electric toothbrushes can also be helpful, since their bristles move at high speeds and are extremely effective at cleaning hard-to-reach areas well. They're a great choice for seniors who might not have a lot of wrist and arm strength to use while brushing—or anyone else who just wants a really strong, effective cleaning every time. Just remember to apply only gentle pressure so you don't hurt your gums.

Of course, just like with cleaning natural teeth, even the most specialized toothbrush can only get you so far. To clean in between your prosthetic teeth and your gums—not to mention your natural teeth and your gums—you need to use dental floss! Flossing should be done at least twice a day, in the morning or at night, and if possible, after every meal. No excuses!

There are cleaning aids that also do wonders, helping to keep your mouth clean and your implants healthy. Water-irrigating devices rinse loosened plaque away from tight spots between teeth. Antibacterial mouth rinses can also go basically anywhere in your mouth, rinse food particles and bacteria away, and add an extra measure of protection. But remember, these are not a substitute for brushing and flossing—that's how you loosen the food particles and bacteria from your teeth in the first place. Whatever other steps you might want to take, brushing and flossing are absolutely essential in order to be sure your new teeth last a lifetime.

Caring for Implant Dentures and Bridges

If your implants support a bridge or denture, cleaning your new teeth might be a little more complicated than what you're used to. For you, the most important area to keep clean will be found under your prosthetic teeth, around the abutments that hold the prosthetics in place, as well as your gums. Floss is the best way to keep these hard-to-reach areas clean. You can squeeze a little toothpaste onto the floss to clean underneath your denture or bridge, running it back and forth to cover the entire length of the device. You can find extra-thick dental floss, which is ideal for this type of cleaning, in your local drugstore.

Professional Care

Now that you have a mouthful of beautiful new teeth, it has never been more important to see your dentist regularly. During the first year of living with your implants, you will likely return for follow-up treatments at least every three months to make sure all is going well. Your dental hygienist will professionally clean your implants and prosthetics, using special plastic scalers (instead of the metal ones used on natural teeth) to remove plaque and tartar without scratching your abutments and a polishing paste designed for prosthetic teeth to keep them shiny and white.

He or she will also make sure you are using the best and most effective methods to take care of your implants on your own. If you're having any problems cleaning your new teeth or aren't sure what to do, your hygienist will work with you to show you how to keep your implants clean.

Your dentist will usually check your implants after your hygienist finishes the cleaning. So if you're experiencing any problems, be sure to tell your hygienist so the dentist will be informed ahead of time.

During your second year with your implants, you will likely be able to drop down to three dental visits a year, or one every four months. And after that, chances are you will see your dentist twice a year, just as you did (or were supposed to do!) when you had your natural teeth.

Of course, if you have any problems at all with your implants or with anything else in your mouth, be sure to let your dentist know right away so that it can be taken care of. Remember, part of having teeth that last a lifetime is taking care of them for a lifetime. If you follow the simple steps outlined here, you should be enjoying your implants for many, many years to come.

Chances are you'll find that caring for your implants really isn't all that different than caring for your natural teeth. Make it a normal part of your daily routine and it will come naturally and easily. Just like the compliments you'll be getting for your beautiful new smile!

So keep eating crunchy apples, keep smiling, keep living, and keep enjoying those beautiful teeth!

The last stories I want to share with you are from Barbara and Grant. Barbara is a determined lady who has a goal of being able to keep all her own teeth (great goal, by the way). And I especially appreciate Grant's words, because he's had experience in the medical field, which makes his comments even more special to me.

Barbara's Story

"I've had trouble with my teeth my entire life. My main goal has always been to keep as many of my teeth as possible.

"I'm seventy-one years old, and a year or so ago, I had to have an implant put in because I had a tooth go bad. It takes several months for the entire process to be completed, but that was no problem at all because I had a temporary tooth during that interim time. One time I was undergoing a surgical procedure (not dental related), and the anesthesiologist commented on how pretty my teeth were. He said he always noticed people's teeth because his wife was a dentist. So I never know where the compliments might come from, but I do know that I have a beautiful set of teeth."

* * *

Grant's Story

"Before I had dental implants, I had a hard time eating, and I wanted to do something about that. I'm glad I did it.

"I had some teeth removed in 2004, and then right afterward I had the implant put in place. I couldn't swallow then, and though the bad teeth didn't show much, the implants probably have improved my self-esteem.

"I knew for a while that I had to do something about my teeth. It wasn't an overnight decision.

"I definitely recommend the dental-implant process to anyone considering it. I think it enabled me to eat properly, and I think it probably extended my lifetime because I can eat better. It increases self-esteem for anyone who has it done. Don't be afraid of it, because it was not nearly as scary as I thought it would be. It was very comfortable, with no pain involved. There's a lot of apprehension in the beginning, but it was just wonderful. I'm so proud I did it."

* * *

ABOUT THE AUTHOR

Dr. Joseph Gaeta, a third-generation Sicilian, grew up in Omaha, Nebraska, where he worked in his parents' restaurant. It was at Gaeta's Restaurant that he learned how to work hard, multitask, and use his hands.

At the ripe old age of six, he began to cook. Dr. Gaeta recalls standing on a milk crate, helping make garlic bread. Even after becoming a dentist and owning his own business, a return home to Omaha and to Gaeta's meant Papa Gaeta would put the doctor to work filling water glasses and waiting tables.

During the 1970s and 1980s, Gaeta's catered to large parties of three hundred and four hundred people. The whole family worked together to make these a success. This is where Dr. Gaeta first learned about serving and taking care of people. As he says, "life is about service."

Dr. Gaeta graduated from Creighton University Dental Board, School of Dental Science, in Omaha. In 1986, he moved to Sarasota, Florida, and opened his practice. Through the years, he has logged over fifteen hundred hours in post-graduate dental-implant education and has been placing and restoring dental implants for over twenty years.

In 1999, Dr. Gaeta achieved board-certification status with the American Board of Oral Implantology/Implant Dentistry (ABOI/ID). Fewer than five hundred dentists worldwide have achieved this status.

Dr. Gaeta is trained in both surgical and restorative technique; he places implants and also restores them to function. There are very few dentists in the United States who do both.

Dr. Gaeta's passion to help others led to his founding of the World Dental Implant Awareness Organization (www.WDIAO.org). The mission of this organization is to create awareness in the world about the devastating consequences of tooth loss and the life changing benefits of dental implants

 As a devotee of health and fitness, Dr. Gaeta is also a triathlete and a marathon runner. He and his son, Joey, love running together and routinely compete in half marathons.

Dr. Gaeta says, "I hope you find this book helpful and informative because dental implants can add *years to your life and life to your years*. And may you have a long, prosperous, healthy life and be able to order any type of meal your heart desires."

Get a free valuable report, *Questions to Ask When Choosing an Implant Dentist,* by visiting **www. yourmissingteetharekillingyou.com.**

May God bless you with the quality of life you deserve.

Take care, and have a blessed day

WARMLY...

Dr.Joseph A Gaeta Jr DDS

REFERENCES

1 Bureau of the Census, "Age and Sex Composition: 2010," by Lindsay M. Howden and Julie A. Meyer, Census Brief (May 2011), http://www.census.gov/prod/cen2010/briefs/c2010br-03.pdf, Fig. 4.

2 Arias, E. "United States Life Tables, 2006," *National Vital Statistics Reports*, vol 58, no 21. Hyattsville, MD: National Center for Health Statistics, 2010.

3 Xu, J. Q., K. D. Kochanek, S. L. Murphy, and B. Tejada-Vera, "Deaths: Final Data for 2007," *National Vital Statistics Reports,* vol 58, no 21. Hyattsville, MD: National Center for Health Statistics, 2010.

4 Vincent, Grayson K., and Victoria A. Velkoff, "The Next Four Decades: The Older Population in the United States 2010 to 2050," Current Population Reports, US Census Bureau, Washington, DC, May 2010, 25–1138.

5 National Center for Chronic Disease Prevention and Health Promotion, Department of Health and Human Services, Centers for Disease Control and Prevention, *Fact Sheet: Oral Health For Adults*, December 2006, Division of Oral Health.

6 National Center for Chronic Disease Prevention and Health Promotion, Department of Health and Human Services, Centers for Disease Control and Prevention, *Fact Sheet: Oral Health for Older Americans*, December 2006, Division Of Oral Health.

7 Centers for Disease Control and Prevention. Surveillance for Dental Caries, Dental Sealants, Tooth Retention, Edentulism, and Enamel Fluorosis. MMWR 2005;54: , 1–44.

8 Dr. Carl Misch, *Rationale for Implant Dentistry*, 8.

9 Axelsson, P., J. Lindhe, and B. Nystrom, "On the Prevention of Cavities and Periodontal Disease: Results of a 15-year Longitudinal Study in Adults," *Journal of Clinical Periodontology* 18 (1991): 182–189.

10 Bodic, F., L. Hamel, E. Lerouxel, M. F. Basle, and D. Chappard, "Bone Loss and Teeth," *Joint Bone Spine* 72 (2005): 215–221.

11 Dr. Carl Misch, *Rationale for Implant Dentistry*, pages 12–15.

12 Mandali, G., I. D. Sener, S. B. Turker, and H. Ulgen, "Factors Affecting the Distribution and Prevalence of Oral Mucosal Lesions in Complete Denture Wearers," *Gerodontology* 28 (2011): 97–103.

13 Gilbert, G. H., R. P. Duncan, M. W. Heft, T. A. Dolan, and W. B. Vogel., "Oral Disadvantage among Dentate Adults," *Community Dentistry and Oral Epidemiology* 25 (1997): 301–313.

14 S. P. Nations et al., "Denture Cream: An Unusual Source of Excess Zinc, Leading to Hypocupremia and Neurologic Disease," *Neurology* 71 (2008): 639–643.

15 Calculations are as follows: Nations and colleagues (2008) reported that the denture cream they tested had between 17 mg and 34 mg of zinc per gram of cream. If the typical tube of denture cream has about 68 grams, then that is at least 1,156 mg per tube.

16 "Zinc," http://ods.od.nih.gov/factsheets/Zinc-QuickFacts.

17 Holm-Pedersen, P., K. Schultz-Larsen, N. Christiansen, and K. Avlund, "Tooth Loss and Subsequent Disability and Mortality in Old Age," *Journal of the American Geriatrics Society* 56 (2008): 429–435.

18 Appollonio, I., C. Carabellese, A. Frattola, and M. Trabucchi, "Dental Status, Quality of Life, and Mortality in an Older Commu-

nity Population: A multivariate approach." *Journal of the American Geriatrics Society* 45 (1997): 1315–1323.

19 Paganini-Hill, A., S. C. White, and K. A. Atchison., "Dental Health Behaviors, Dentition, and Mortality in the Elderly: The Leisure World Cohort Study," *Journal of Aging Research* 2011 (2011): 1–10.

20 R. Touger-Decker, R. D. Sirois, and C. C. Mobley, *Nutrition and Oral Medicine* (Totowa, New Jersey: Humana Press, 2005).

21 Sheiham, A., J. Steele, W. Marcenes, S. Finch, and A. Walls, "The Relationship between Oral Health Status and Body Mass Index among Older People: A National Survey of Older People in Great Britain," *British Dental Journal* 192 (2002).

22 Sullivan, D. H., and Walls, R. C., "Protein-energy Undernutrition and the Risk of Mortality within Six Years of Hospital Discharge," *Journal of the American College of Nutrition* 17 (1998): 571–578.

A portion of the proceeds from the book *Your Missing Teeth Are Killing You!* are donated to the World Dental Implant Awareness Organization

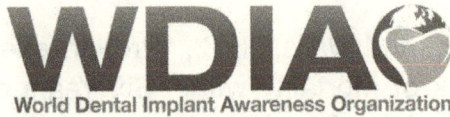

World Dental Implant Awareness Organization

The mission of WDIAO is to create world awareness about the devastating consequences of tooth loss, the life changing benefits of dental implants, as well as serve select individuals in need. To learn more on how you can help support WDIAO, or for more information please visit:

www.WDIAO.org

www.ingramcontent.com/pod-product-compliance
Lightning Source LLC
Chambersburg PA
CBHW030024290326
41934CB00005B/473